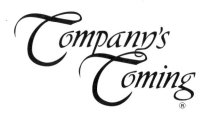

# Gluten-free Cooking

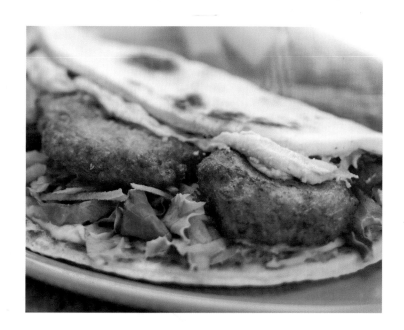

Ted Wolff

**Cover image:** Veggie Calzone, see page 136

First Printing May 2013

**Library and Archives Canada Cataloguing in Publication**

Wolff, Ted

Gluten-free cooking / Ted Wolff.

(Healthy cooking series)

Includes index.

ISBN 978-1-927126-41-7

1. Gluten-free diet--Recipes.  2. Cookbooks  I. Title.

II. Series: Healthy cooking series

RM237.86.W655 2013          641.5′638        C2012-906344-4

Published by

**Company's Coming Publishing Limited**

2311 – 96 Street NW

Edmonton, Alberta, Canada T6N 1G3

Tel: 780-450-6223   Fax: 780-450-1857

www.companyscoming.com

Company's Coming is a registered trademark owned by Company's Coming Publishing Limited

We acknowledge the financial support of the Government of Canada through the Canada Book Fund for our publishing activities.

Printed in China

*PC:*16

# CONTENTS

Introduction...............................................................5

Basic Recipes...........................................................9

Appetizers and Snacks.............................................10

Soups and Salads....................................................32

Mains • Beef.............................................................50

Mains • Chicken.......................................................72

Mains • Turkey.........................................................94

Mains • Fish and Seafood........................................98

Mains • Pork and Lamb..........................................110

Mains • Vegetarian................................................128

Sides......................................................................142

Sauces...................................................................154

Index......................................................................158

Acknowledgements................................................160

# The Company's Coming Legacy

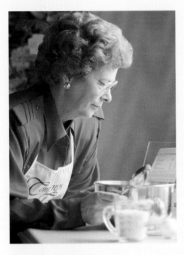

Jean Paré grew up with an understanding that family, friends and home cooking are the key ingredients for a good life. A busy mother of four, Jean developed a knack for creating quick and easy recipes using everyday ingredients. For 18 years, she operated a successful catering business from her home kitchen in the small prairie town of Vermilion, Alberta, Canada. During that time, she earned a reputation for great food, courteous service and reasonable prices. Steadily increasing demand for her recipes led to the founding of Company's Coming Publishing Limited in 1981.

The first Company's Coming cookbook, *150 Delicious Squares*, was an immediate bestseller. As more titles were introduced, the company quickly earned the distinction of publishing Canada's most popular cookbooks. Company's Coming continues to gain new supporters in Canada, the United States and throughout the world by adhering to Jean's Golden Rule of Cooking: Never share a recipe you wouldn't use yourself. It's an approach that has worked—millions of times over!

A familiar and trusted name in the kitchen, Company's Coming has extended its reach throughout the home with other types of books and products for everyday living.

Though humble about her achievements, Jean Paré is one of North America's most loved and recognized authors. The recipient of many awards, Jean was appointed Member of the Order of Canada, her country's highest lifetime achievement honour.

Today, Jean Paré's influence as founding author, mentor and moral compass is evident in all aspects of the company she founded. Every recipe created and every product produced upholds the family values and work ethic she instilled. Readers the world over will continue to be encouraged and inspired by her legacy for generations to come.

## *Nutrition Information Guidelines*

Each recipe is analyzed using the most current version of the Canadian Nutrient File from Health Canada, which is based on the United States Department of Agriculture (USDA) Nutrient Database.

- If more than one ingredient is listed (such as "butter or hard margarine"), or if a range is given (1 – 2 tsp., 5 – 10 mL), only the first ingredient or first amount is analyzed.

- For meat, poultry and fish, the serving size per person is based on the recommended 4 oz. (113 g) uncooked weight (without bone), which is 2 – 3 oz. (57 – 85 g) cooked weight (without bone)— approximately the size of a deck of playing cards.

- Milk used is 1% M.F. (milk fat), unless otherwise stated.

- Cooking oil used is canola oil, unless otherwise stated.

- Ingredients indicating "sprinkle," "optional," or "for garnish" are not included in the nutrition information.

- The fat in recipes and combination foods can vary greatly depending on the sources and types of fats used in each specific ingredient. For these reasons, the amount of saturated, monounsaturated and polyunsaturated fats may not add up to the total fat content.

# Introduction

## Gluten-free Cooking? Isn't that just Meat and Potatoes?

I've heard this question many times, and anyone with a gluten intolerance will have experienced times at a party, a restaurant or a family gathering when that was indeed all that was left on the plate—a plain piece of meat and some plain potatoes without sauce, gravy or dip.

Whether you are on a gluten-free diet or are preparing a meal for a friend or loved one, this book offers easy and well-tested gluten-free recipes for some quick meals, as well as some for a more elaborate gourmet dinner.

It is true that you can survive on just plain meat and potatoes for a while, but that would be a rather bland-tasting diet after a while. Gluten-free cooking offers us a renewed opportunity to pay attention to how we view our food and eating habits, and ultimately puts us back in charge of what we put into our bodies. As we are exploring ingredients and alternatives to gluten-rich flours and starches in many main dishes, appetizers, sauces and side dishes, we are embarking on an exploration of tastes, textures and senses, be it by ourselves or with friends and families. Nothing tastes better than homemade gluten-free tortellini or gluten-free perogies served with some tasty gluten-free bruschetta or gluten-free garlic toast. It is time to get off Facebook, turn of the computer, silence the cell phone and get cooking.

## Observations from a Yodelling Gluten-free Master

As discussed in my first book published by Company's Coming, *Gluten-free Baking*, I like to emphasize that your primary focus in living gluten-free is to assure a safe supply of ingredients from dedicated gluten-free sources. There are many specialty gluten-free suppliers out there. If you're in doubt, ask.

Gluten is a cereal protein that can cause various negative health issues to those who are intolerant to this protein or any portion of it. In the context of this book, *gluten-free* refers to the absence of any wheat, barley, rye, oats, spelt, kamut, triticale or any derivatives thereof. A gluten-free diet is currently the only acceptable choice for anyone with celiac disease or who is in any way intolerant of gluten.

Just like in any type of gluten-free food preparation, at home or elsewhere, you need to watch what you're eating. **Avoid:** wheat, barley, rye, oats, spelt, kamut, triticale and derivatives.

As alternatives to the above no-nos on a gluten-free diet, use a variety of other gluten-free ingredients. **Embrace:** white long-grain rice flour, millet flour, wild rice flour, Montina grass, buckwheat, chia, amaranth, quinoa, teff, sorghum, white corn flour, popcorn flour, saba flour, yellow corn flour, white medium-grain rice flour, cornmeal, tapioca starch, arrowroot starch, potato starch, pea starch, brown rice, pea fibres, whole bean flour, garbanzo bean flour, fava bean flour, red rice, almond meal, hazelnut flour, sweet rice flour, almond flour, lupine flour, chestnut flour, flax meal, potato flour, etc...

Make sure the sources of your gluten-free ingredients provide a guaranteed gluten-free environment.

Now, after you've spent your valuable money on gluten-free ingredients, ensure that they they are not going to end up cross-contaminated at home. You've gone to the trouble of getting gluten-free supplies and bringing them to your kitchen— and then you try to cook gluten-free products in the same space where the counters are sprinkled with fine wheat flour, or maybe some wheat crumbs are still stuck to your family's pots and pans. No, no, not a good idea. It also defeats the purpose if you store your gluten-free treasures right next to supplies that contain gluten.

Let's say all these issues are dealt with and there is no wheat flour and no cross-contamination. But your friend or mom just finished cooking some fresh wheat tortellini from the local Italian shop, straining them through your only colander? Better have all of these cleaned up and washed once again before starting with your own tasty gluten-free tortellini. I know that it sounds a bit silly, but you know that I am right. If you're the one cooking for a family member or friend who is on a gluten-free diet, be very diligent with your kitchen environment. Keep your gluten-free space, storage and utensils separate. Your loved one will thank you.

As far as cooking goes, try to free yourself from the idea that you can only cook something if you have all the ingredients that the recipe calls for on hand. Be creative; be bold. If you're missing one starch in the recipe, replace it with a different starch or a gluten-free flour. Making a gluten-free pasta using a variation of other gluten-free starches than what is called for in the recipe, or making a pastry dough with a little bit more potato starch then corn starch, will still be nice and tasty. Experiment if you are out of one ingredient or have a hard time sourcing it. Just be sure to always write down what you do. You just never know when you'll come up with a winning recipe. Also, there are never any mistakes. There are some ingredients that will give you better results, and if you can, you will find it beneficial to stick to the recipes that get the best results— but a gravy will still be a great gravy regardless of whether you use potato starch or sweet rice flour.

There are many great sources that deal in detail with gluten-free diets, hidden sources of gluten and specific gluten-free products— books, websites, brochures, chat groups, online forums, blogs and more. The following list of ingredients looks specifically at the gluten-free products you'll encounter in this book. Living gluten-free does not have to be a hardship when you can still enjoy delicious food!

# Glossary of Ingredients

**Almond flour:** Almonds ground into fine flour, either blanched or brown. I prefer brown myself.

**Ascorbic acid:** One form of vitamin C. In the dough improver recipe (page 9), we use a powdered form. Ascorbic acid can be helpful as a dough strengthener and helps to create a finer crumb structure. You will find it either as "Ascorbic Acid" or "Powdered Vitamin C" in many natural food stores, grocery stores or bulk food stores.

**Baking powder:** Most North American baking powders are now gluten-free and use corn starch as the carrier for the leavening ingredients. I did develop a specific gluten-free baking powder a few years ago and it is sold now under the brand name KinnActive through Kinnikinnick Foods. For the purpose of this book, a gluten-free grocery brand (such as Magic) was used.

**Brown rice flour:** Ground from rice that still has the endosperm and bran. The brown rice flour used in these recipes is stabilized, meaning the flour can be stored at room temperatures.

**Buckwheat flour:** Of course this flour has nothing to do with bucks or wheat at all. In fact, it is not a grain at all but is related to the rhubarb family. There are two main types of buckwheat flour. The first is milled from roasted buckwheat (kasha), which is dark in colour and has a strong flavour. The second is ground from unroasted buckwheat and provides for a milder flavour. I use both. I like buckwheat for its high nutritional values and its taste.

**Butter:** In most cases, salted butter is implied.

**Cornmeal:** Made from corn. I use very fine cornmeal, mainly for dusting purposes.

**Cornstarch:** Made from corn. A tasteless starch commonly used in gluten-free baking to lighten texture.

**Dough improver (see page 9):** A very simple mix of 3 ingredients (powdered lecithin, ginger and ascorbic acid), which you can make yourself. It gives a little punch to your yeast and final product.

**Eggs:** Use organic large eggs; the chickens and your well-being will be thankful. Use at room temperature whenever possible. Room temperature eggs are easier to incorporate into your batter, the egg whites will produce a larger volume and, in yeast-risen recipes, will not cool down the dough too much. To get eggs to room temperature quickly, take them out of the fridge and place in hot water for 10 minutes.

**Egg whites:** While making recipes calling for egg whites, keep in mind that you will have leftover egg yolks. You could use the egg yolks in the doughnut recipes (published in *Gluten-free Baking*) or the Tortellini recipe (see page 92), which call only for egg yolks.

**Gluten-free all-purpose flour (see page 9):** This gluten-free all-purpose flour combines specific ingredients to address thickening-texturizing as well as freeze-thaw stability in the recipes.

**Gluten-free pasta:** Depending where you live and which stores you frequent to source your gluten-free supplies, you will encounter many choices for gluten-free pasta nowadays. Even regular grocery stores will stock at least rice pastas and corn pastas from various brands. Although the ingredients might be the same in some "Asian-style" pasta (rice sticks, etc.) and the more "Western-style" pasta (penne, lasagna, etc.), the latter is typically processed in a way to duplicate its wheat counterpart. Experiment with different brands, and if you are lucky enough to get your hands on some more specialty formulated "Italian-style" pasta from Europe, go try them. Some recipes go better with a corn pasta, where in others the plain taste of rice-based ones is favored by cooks. Tinkyada, Rizopia, Bi-Aglut, Polial, Aglutin, Aproten, Pastariso, Farabella, Le Veneziane, Felicia are just some of the many brands available. Try the gluten-free pasta recipes in this book to taste heavenly tortellini and ravioli (see page 92).

**Granulated soy or rice lecithin:** In the dough improver recipe (see page 9), lecithin is used in its powdered form and acts as an emulsifier to improve the texture and quality of baked products. It is widely available in many health food stores, your local grocery market or online.

**Guar gum:** A potential alternative to xanthan gum, but with different texturizing characteristics than xanthan gum. Some people use it directly to replace xanthan gum, which I find in many recipes somewhat too gummy. In some recipes, though, xanthan gum and guar gum work well if used together. Guar gum is also being reported as having laxative effects for some people.

**Masa harina corn flour:** Lime-treated white maize/corn flour. Mainly used for tortillas. It is different from yellow cornflour, which is simply ground corn kernels.

**Mirin:** Mirin is a Japanese seasoning used only for cooking. It is derived from distilled sake, which is put through a brewing process in combination with sticky sweet rice and a special yeast. Mirin is slightly sweet, but cannot be consumed as a beverage. Sake can be used in cooking as well, but it is much better consumed as a beverage.

**Paprika:** There are two types of parika used in this book: regular paprika and Hungarian paprika. Hungarian paprika is slightly sweeter and in most cases darker in colour with a stronger flavour profile.

**Pea fibre III:** A natural food-grade vegetable fibre manufactured from the hulls of Canadian yellow peas. This fibre is gluten-, lactose- and cholesterol-free. It provides a great source of insoluble fibre fortification. **Substitution:** Pea fibre III can be replaced by cellulose fibre or soy fibre. If none of these fibres are available to you, leave out the pea fibre and reduce the liquids by about 2–3 Tbsp per Tbsp of fibre used.

**Pea fibre 80:** A food-grade vegetable fibre that offers both nutrition and functionality due to its high level of soluble and insoluble fibres. It improves texture, mouth-feel and freeze–thaw stability. **Substitution:** Pea fibre 80 can be replaced by 1/2 the amount cellulose fibre or soy fibre and 1/2 the amount inulin fibre or psyllium husk powder. If none of these fibres are available to you, leave out the pea fibre and reduce the liquids by about 2–3 Tbsp per Tbsp of fibre used.

**Pea protein:** Natural food-grade pea proteins offer a high level of nutrition. Pea protein is composed of an excellent amino acid profile and is absent in gluten, lactose, cholesterol and anti-nutritional factors. **Substitution:** Pea protein can be substituted by soy protein, rice protein or isolated whey protein.

**Pea starch:** A native starch made from Canadian yellow field peas. A wonderful alternative to other gluten-free starches. Very unique functionality and high water binding capacity. Provides baked goods with larger volume. This starch is high in slow-digested starch components that provide a slower release of carbohydrates than other starches. **Substitution:** Pea starch can be replaced by a mixture of potato, corn and tapioca starch, using an equal 1/3 amount of each.

**Potato starch:** Made from potatoes. Increases volume due to its larger particle size. Can be replaced by pea starch, but use about 20% less of the pea starch.

**Rice vinegar:** Rice vinegar is a staple seasoning in many dishes with an Eastern influence. It is slightly less acidic than white vinegar. It will add the sour note to many sweet-and-sour dishes and finds a use in many sushi dishes as well.

**Sweet rice flour:** Also called sticky or glutinous, rice flour is made from sweet rice, which provides a more sticky batter and in the right combination adds a moisture-enhancing component to your baked goods. Sweet rice flour is also freeze–thaw stable, meaning if used in pie fillings and so on the food will not separate on reheating or refreezing.

**Tamari sauce:** Traditonally, tamari sauce was always just made from soybeans and is believed to have originated from Japan. However, make sure to always check as there are some soy sauces labelled tamari that may contain wheat. Tamari is somewhat stronger in flavour and darker in colour compared to soy sauce, which is typically made from soybeans and some sort of grain. Make sure any soy sauce you are cooking with has only gluten-free ingredients.

**Tapioca starch:** A fine white root starch. Gives baked goods a light and chewy texture.

**White rice flour:** Ground from rice that has the endosperm, bran and hull removed. There are various types of rice used for white rice flour, including medium rice and long-grain rice. If you have access to medium rice flour, go get it.

**Xanthan gum:** One of the most-used texturizing agents used in gluten-free baking. Basically it works by binding the liquids and dry ingredients into a matrix that provides structure during baking. There are several grades of xanthan gums being sold, each with their own binding capacity. For this book, a powdered xanthan gum was used (instead of a granular type). Depending on the binding capacity, you might have to experiment with the amounts you use in each recipe.

**Yeast:** In most cases traditional active dry yeast is used. There are numerous options for yeast nowadays. You could substitute instant (quick-rise) yeast, but keep in mind that you need to add the extra sugar back into the dry mix. Also, instant yeast will require very warm liquid and a warm batter temperature to work well. It will cut down on leavening time. Wherever available, fresh yeast is wonderful to use for leavening power and flavour. Fresh yeast goes straight into the dough.

**Yellow corn flour:** Ground from regular yellow corn. Used in combination with other flours, it adds a nice colour and texture component. Differs from masa harina as it is not treated with lime and does not work as well in tortillas.

## Basic Recipes

It is best to store the gluten-free all-purpose flour in an airtight container (plastic, glass or metal) at room temperature (between 16 to 25°C, if possible). Its shelf life depends somewhat on age of sourced ingredients, but typically should last a minimum of 12 months.

The dough improver should be kept in an airtight container and, for extended storage duration, should be kept in the fridge. You might consider using a quarter or half the recipe if you're not planning on doing too much baking.

# Gluten-free All-purpose Flour

**Makes 6 cups**

A very basic gluten-free flour/starch combination that you can use as a one-for-one flour substitute in most recipes. This combination provides both thickening qualities as well as some freeze–thaw stability. Adjust the amount of all-purpose flour used in each recipe according to desired consistency.

**2 cups (500 mL) white rice flour**

**1 cup (250 mL) pea starch**

**1 cup (250 mL) potato starch**

**1 cup (250 mL) sweet rice flour**

**1/2 cup (125 mL) cornstarch**

**1/2 cup (125 mL) tapioca starch**

**1 Tbsp (15 mL) guar gum**

**1 Tbsp (15 mL) xanthan gum**

Mix all ingredients together and store in an airtight container.

# Dough Improver

**Makes about 2 cups**

This "baker's little helper" gives some extra punch to your yeast and improves breadcrumb structure.

**2 cups (500 mL) granulated soy or rice lecithin**

**1 Tbsp (15 mL) ascorbic acid**

**1 Tbsp (15 mL) powdered ginger**

Mix granulated lecithin in a blender to achieve a more powdery consistency. Then mix all ingredients well and store in a sealable container. Use 1 to 1 1/2 tsp (5 to 7 mL) per loaf of bread or according to recipe.

# Gluten-free French Bread

**Makes 1 loaf**

A slightly denser and chewier quality makes this bread great for French toast. The omission of oil is not an oversight.

**1/4 cup (60 mL) warm water**

**1 Tbsp (15 mL) active dry yeast**

**2 tsp (10 mL) sugar**

**1 1/2 cups (375 mL) tapioca starch**

**1 1/2 cups (375 mL) white rice flour**

**1/4 cup (60 mL) whey powder**

**2 Tbsp (30 mL) pea fibre 80**

**2 Tbsp (30 mL) sugar**

**4 tsp (20 mL) xanthan gum**

**1 tsp (5 mL) dough improver (see left column)**

**1 tsp (5 mL) salt**

**1 3/4 cups (425 mL) water**

**1/4 cup (125 mL) egg whites, room temperature**

Place first 3 ingredients in a small bowl.

Mix next 8 ingredients in a large bowl.

Mix water and egg whites in a separate bowl. Add egg white mixture and yeast mixture to flour mixture. Mix until a smooth batter is formed. Pour batter into greased 9 x 5 inch (23 x 12.5 inch) baking pan and smooth with a wet spatula. Place in a warm place and cover with a damp towel. Let rise until doubled in size. Place pans in a 350°F (175°C) oven on middle rack. Bake for 50 minutes until bread sounds hollow when tapped on bottom. Place on a wire rack to cool.

*1 loaf: 1879 Calories; 6 g Total Fat (0 g Mono, 0 g Poly, 1 g Sat); 30 mg Cholesterol; 415 g Carbohydrate; 35 g Fibre; 46 g Protein; 2868 mg Sodium*

# Spicy Cheddar Spritz

## Makes 9 dozen

A nice spicy cheese hors d'oeuvre that will store well—but most likely it will be gone before the party has even started.

**1 1/2 to 1 3/4 cups (375 to 425 mL) gluten-free all-purpose flour (see page 9)**

**1 1/2 tsp (7 mL) Hungarian paprika**

**1/2 tsp (2 mL) cayenne pepper**

**1/2 cup (125 mL) butter**

**1 lb (454 g) finely grated sharp Cheddar cheese**

Preheat oven to 375°F (190°C). Mix first 3 ingredients in a small bowl. Set aside.

With a mixer, beat butter until softened. Slowly add cheese, beating well after each addition. With mixer running, add flour mixture in 4 additions, beating well after each addition. Spoon into pastry bag fitted with a star (#7) tip. Pipe batter onto parchment paper–lined baking sheet into 2-inch (5 cm) circles or 2- to 3-inch (5 to 7.5 cm) long ovals. Bake in preheated oven for 12 to 15 minutes until light brown.

*1 hors d'oeuvre: 31 Calories; 2 g Total Fat (0 g Mono, 0 g Poly, 1 g Sat); 7 mg Cholesterol; 1 g Carbohydrate; 0 g Fibre; 0 g Protein; 34 mg Sodium*

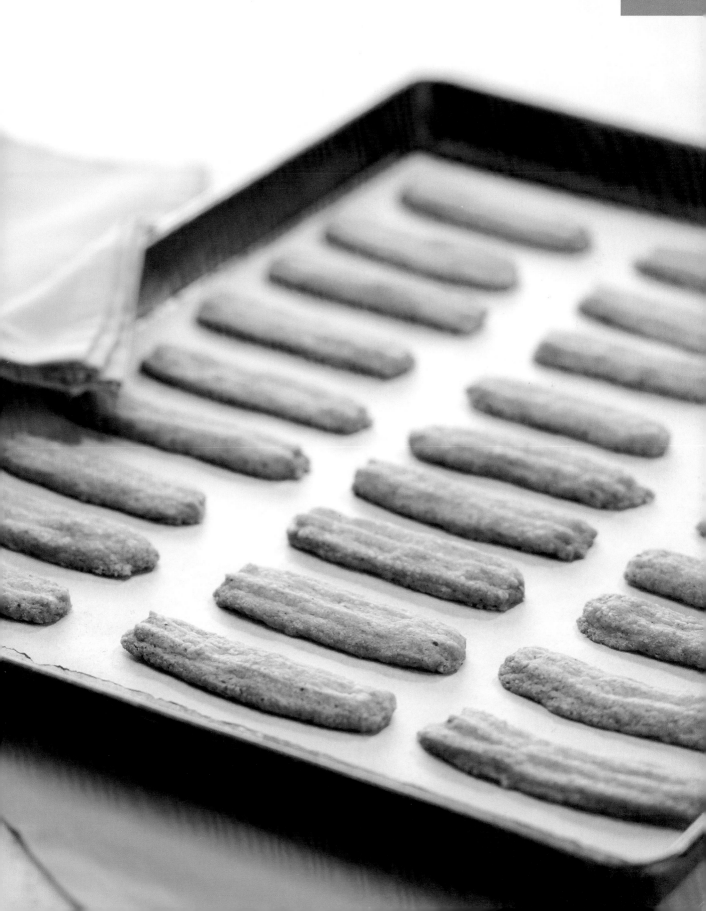

# Shrimp Tartlets

## Makes about 18

Great as an appetizer as well as a snack or meal, these seafood tartlets can be cooked in the prepared tartlet shells or without pastry in greased tart pans.

### Tartlet Shells

1 cup (250 mL) white rice flour

1/2 cup (125 mL) sweet rice flour

1/2 cup (125 mL) tapioca starch

1/4 cup (60 mL) pea starch

1 Tbsp (15 mL) pea fibre 80

1 Tbsp (15 mL) sugar

1 1/2 tsp (7 mL) xanthan gum

1 tsp (5 mL) baking powder

1 tsp (5 mL) salt

3/4 cup (175 mL) lard (or shortening)

1 large egg, fork-beaten

2 Tbsp (30 mL) cold water, approximately

2 Tbsp (30 mL) vinegar

*(continued on next page)*

**Tartlet Shells:** Combine first 9 ingredients in a large bowl. Cut in lard until mixture resembles coarse crumbs.

Add egg, water and vinegar. Stir until mixture starts to come together. Do not over mix. Dust hands with sweet rice flour. Turn out pastry onto work surface covered with parchment paper. Divide pastry into 2 portions. Shape each portion into slightly flattened disc. Roll out each portion to about 1/8 inch (3 mm) thickness. Cut out circles with 3-inch (7.5 cm) round cookie cutter. Press into small tart pans.

**Shrimp Filling:** Preheat oven to 350°F (175°C). If making tartlets without shells, grease 12 tart pans. Mix first 3 ingredients in a medium bowl. Divide shrimp mixture evenly among tart pans.

Whisk eggs and sour cream in a separate medium bowl. Pour into each cup until shrimp mixture is just covered. Sprinkle seafood seasoning over top. Bake in preheated oven for 20 to 25 minutes until knife inserted in centre of tartlet comes out clean.

*1 tartlet: 248 Calories; 17 g Total Fat (1 g Mono, 0.5 g Poly, 8 g Sat); 127 mg Cholesterol; 14 g Carbohydrate; 1 g Fibre; 9 g Protein; 290 mg Sodium*

*(continued on next page)*

**Swiss Cheese Tartlets:** Omit shrimp, peppers and cheese. Replace with 1 cup (250 mL) *each* of cubed ham, finely chopped pineapple and grated Swiss cheese.

**Chicken Tartlets:** Omit shrimp, peppers and cheese. Replace with 1 cup (250 mL) *each* of chopped cooked chicken, finely chopped portobello mushrooms and grated Gruyère (or medium Cheddar) cheese.

## Shrimp Filling

**1 cup (250 mL) chopped cooked shrimp (peeled and de-veined)**

**1 cup (250 mL) finely chopped bell peppers**

**1 cup (250 mL) grated medium Cheddar cheese**

**8 large eggs, fork-beaten**

**1/3 cup (75 mL) sour cream**

**seafood seasoning, to taste**

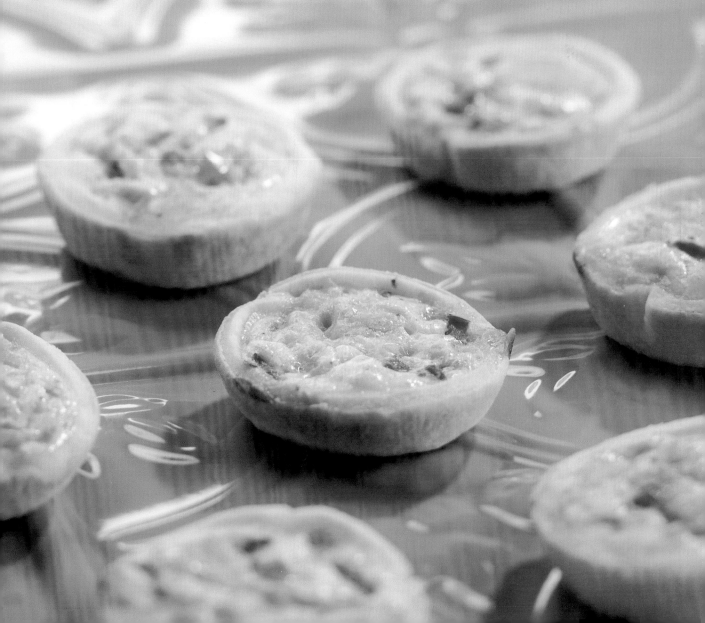

# Puff Shrimp with Orange Ginger Sauce

## Makes about 7 dozen

These versatile offerings are great as a side dish, appetizer or snack if you're not afraid of fried food. Keep in mind that they do contain alcohol. The orange and ginger flavour combination really hits the spot.

**lard, shortening or cooking oil, for deep frying**

### Orange Ginger Sauce

**1 1/2 cup (375 mL) orange marmalade**

**1/3 cup (75 mL) medium sherry**

**3 Tbsp (45 mL) soy sauce**

**1 1/2 pieces of ginger root, 1/2 to 1 inch (1.2 to 2.5 cm) length**

**1 garlic clove, minced**

### Batter

**3/4 to 1 cup (175 to 250 mL) gluten-free all-purpose flour (see page 9)**

**1 1/2 tsp (7 mL) salt**

**1/4 to 1/2 tsp (1 to 2 mL) pepper**

**5 egg yolks, fork-beaten**

**3/4 cup (175 mL) white wine**

**5 egg whites, fork-beaten**

**3 lbs (1.4 kg) uncooked medium shrimp (peeled and de-veined)**

Heat lard in deep fryer to 350°F (175°C) according to manufacturer's instructions.

**Orange Ginger Sauce:** Heat all 5 ingredients in a small saucepan on medium for 3 to 4 minutes until bubbles form around edge of saucepan. Remove from heat. Remove and discard ginger. Cover to keep warm.

**Batter:** Mix flour, salt and pepper in a medium bowl. Add egg yolks and white wine, stirring constantly. Add egg whites and mix well.

Dip shrimp in batter. Deep-fry, in batches, in hot lard for about 3 minutes per batch until golden brown and cooked through. Transfer to paper towel–lined plate to drain. Serve shrimp with orange ginger dipping sauce.

*1 shrimp: 58 Calories; 2 g Total Fat (0 g Mono, 0 g Poly, 0 g Sat); 38 mg Cholesterol; 5 g Carbohydrate; 0 g Fibre; 4 g Protein; 106 mg Sodium*

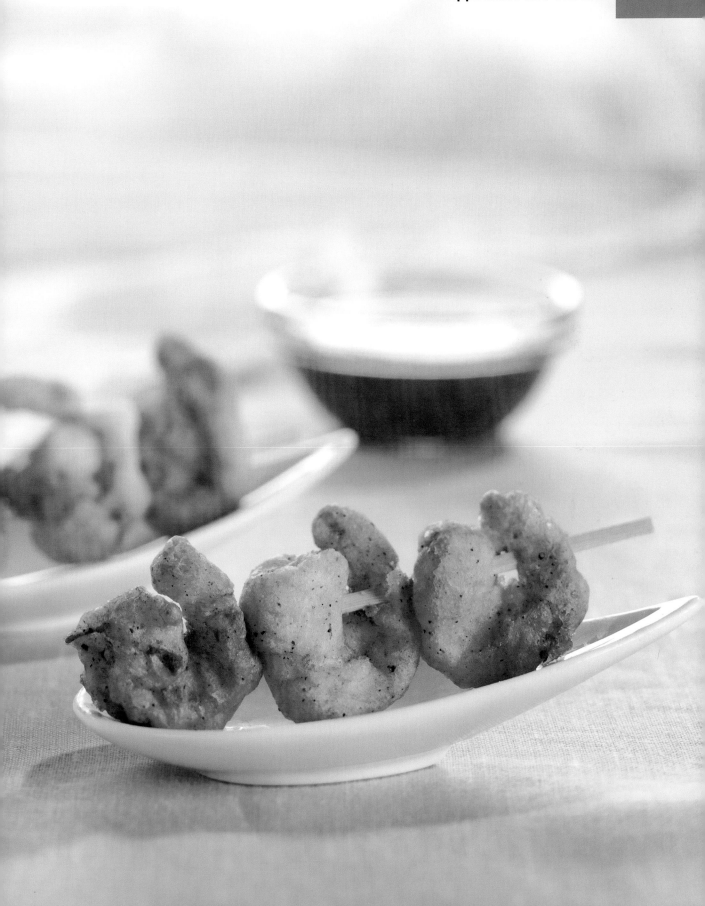

# Bruschetta

## Serves 6 to 8

A toasted, golden brown, French-style bread seasoned with olive oil and topped with fresh plum tomatoes and aromatic basil. You can use the bread recipe below or use any other gluten-free baguettes or French bread.

## Bread

1/4 cup (60 mL) warm water

2 tsp (10 mL) active dry yeast

2 tsp (10 mL) sugar

1 1/8 cups (280 mL) pea starch

3/4 cup (175 mL) tapioca starch

1/4 cup (60 mL) whey powder

1 Tbsp (15 mL) pea fibre 80

2 tsp (10 mL) baking powder

2 tsp (10 mL) xanthan gum

1 tsp (5 mL) dough improver (see page 9)

1 tsp (5 mL) salt

1 tsp (5 mL) sugar

1 1/4 cup (300 mL) water

1/4 cup (60 mL) cooking oil

1 egg white, room temperature

*(continued on next page)*

**Bread:** Place first 3 ingredients in a small bowl. Let stand for 10 minutes until foamy.

Mix next 9 ingredients in a large bowl.

Mix remaining 3 ingredients in a separate bowl. Add egg mixture and yeast mixture to starch mixture. Stir until a smooth batter is formed. Pour batter into a greased 9 x 5 inch (23 x 12.5 cm) baking pan. Smooth with a wet spatula. Place in a warm place and cover with a damp towel. Let rise until about doubled in size. Place pan in 350°F (175°C) oven on middle rack and bake for about 45 to 50 minutes until bread sounds hollow when tapped. Place on a wire rack to cool. Once bread is cooled, slice bread diagonally into 1-inch (2.5 cm) slices. Place on an ungreased baking sheet. Bake in 350°F (175°C) oven for 10 to 20 minutes until slightly golden.

**Topping:** Combine all 7 ingredients in a medium bowl. Scoop topping onto toasted bread slices and serve.

*1 serving: 292 Calories; 12 g Total Fat (8 g Mono, 3 g Poly, 1 g Sat); 5 mg Cholesterol; 44 g Carbohydrate; 4 g Fibre; 5 g Protein; 539 mg Sodium*

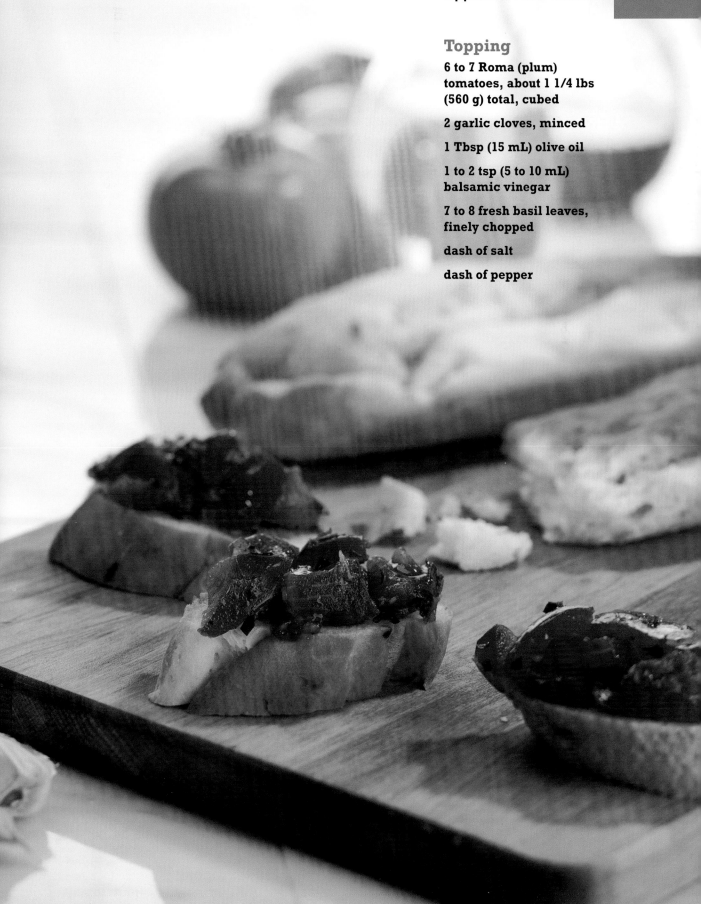

## Topping

**6 to 7 Roma (plum)
tomatoes, about 1 1/4 lbs
(560 g) total, cubed**

**2 garlic cloves, minced**

**1 Tbsp (15 mL) olive oil**

**1 to 2 tsp (5 to 10 mL)
balsamic vinegar**

**7 to 8 fresh basil leaves,
finely chopped**

**dash of salt**

**dash of pepper**

# Green Onion Cakes

## Makes about 15

A staple at any festival or outdoor event, these flat, pan-fried cakes are easy to make. Serve them as a side dish or make them into a meal on their own. I dip them in balsamic vinegar, but you can try any sauce you'd like.

**2/3 cup (150 mL) sweet rice flour**

**2/3 cup (150 mL) tapioca starch**

**1/3 cup (75 mL) pea starch**

**2 Tbsp (30 mL) sugar**

**2 Tbsp (30 mL) whey powder**

**1 1/2 Tbsp (25 mL) active dry yeast**

**1 1/2 Tbsp (25 mL) pea fibre III**

**2 tsp (10 mL) xanthan gum**

**1 1/4 tsp (6 mL) guar gum**

**1/4 tsp (1 mL) salt**

*(continued on next page)*

Mix first 10 ingredients in a medium metal bowl.

Mix next 4 ingredients in a separate bowl. Add egg mixture to flour mixture. Knead together or use a heavy-duty mixer with a dough hook attachment until combined. Mix in green onion. Turn out dough onto surface lightly dusted with sweet rice flour. Divide dough into 2 to 3 inch (5 to 7.5 cm) balls. Roll dough pieces out in rounds to 1/2 inch (12 mm) thickness. Place on a greased baking sheet. Place in a warm place and cover with a damp towel. Let rise for 15 to 20 minutes.

Heat large frying pan on medium. Add 1 to 2 Tbsp (15 to 30 mL) cooking oil. Cook green onion cakes in batches for 4 to 5 minutes on each side until golden brown. Add more cooking oil between batches if necessary to prevent sticking. Serve green onion cakes hot with chosen dipping sauce.

*1 cake: 109 Calories; 5 g Total Fat (3 g Mono, 1 g Poly, 0 g Sat); 10 mg Cholesterol; 15 g Carbohydrate; 2 g Fibre; 2 g Protein; 60 mg Sodium*

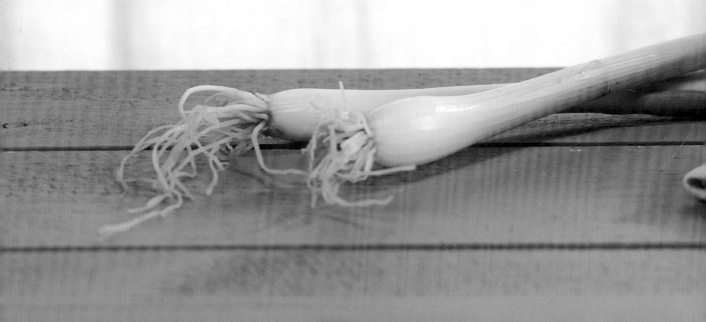

1/2 cup (125 mL) water

3 Tbsp (45 mL) cooking oil

1 large egg, room temperature

1 egg white (large), room temperature

6 to 8 green onions, cut into 1/4 inch (6 mm) pieces

2 to 4 Tbsp (30 to 60 mL) cooking oil, *divided*

1/4 cup (60 mL) balsamic vinegar or gluten-free teriyaki sauce (see page 156), optional

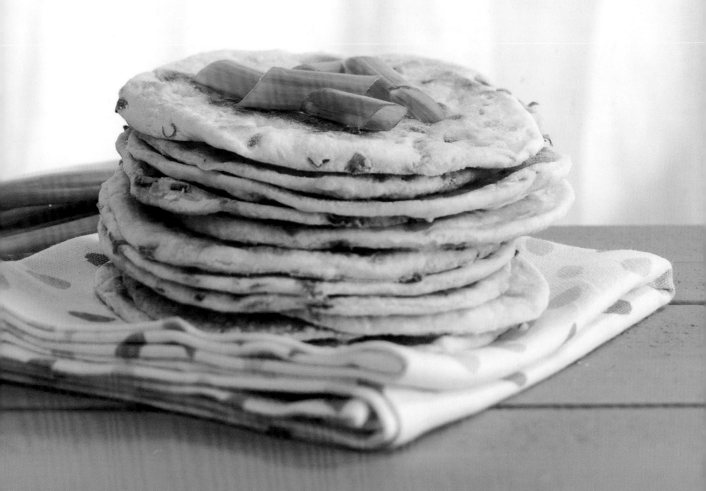

# Corn Dogs

## Makes 8

This famous staple of fairgrounds combines fried dough with a wiener on a stick, somewhat like a sausage in a blanket with the typical corn batter.

**lard, for deep-frying**

Heat lard in deep fryer to 350°F (175°C) according to manufacturer's instructions.

**6 egg whites (large)**

Beat egg whites until stiff.

**1/2 cup (125 mL) milk**

**1/2 cup (125 mL) canned kernel corn, drained and finely chopped**

**1/4 cup (60 mL) cream-style corn**

**1/4 cup (60 mL) cooking oil**

Mix next 4 ingredients in a separate bowl. Add cornbread and muffin mix in 3 additions, mixing well after each addition. Slowly fold corn mixture into egg whites until no white streaks remain. Do not beat or over mix.

**1 1/2 cup (375 mL) gluten-free cornbread and muffin mix (such as Kinnikinnick brand, or see Tip, page 21)**

Push a wooden stick through the length of each wiener. Dip in corn batter. Deep-fry, in batches, in hot cooking oil for 2 to 3 minutes until golden brown. Remove and place on paper towels to drain.

**8 large gluten-free wieners**

*1 corn dog: 372 Calories; 23 g Total Fat (5 g Mono, 2 g Poly, 6 g Sat); 44 mg Cholesterol; 32 g Carbohydrate; 1 g Fibre; 10 g Protein; 780 mg Sodium*

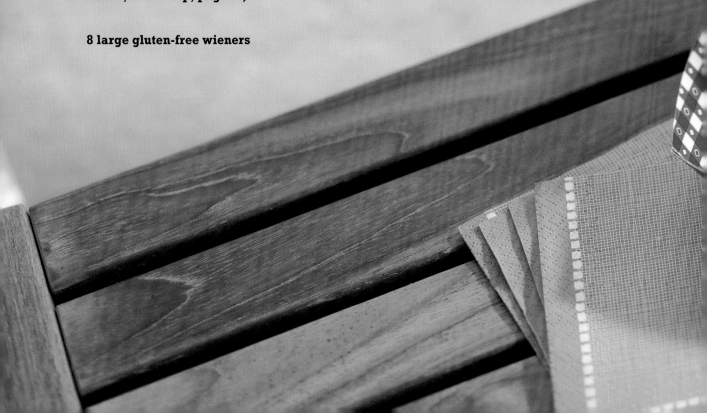

## Tip

Instead of using store-bought cornbread and muffin mix, you can make your own. Combine 3/4 cup (175 mL) gluten-free all-purpose flour (see page 9), 3/4 cup (175 mL) fine cornmeal, 1/4 cup (60 mL) sugar, 2 1/4 tsp (11 mL) baking powder and 3/4 tsp (4 mL) salt.

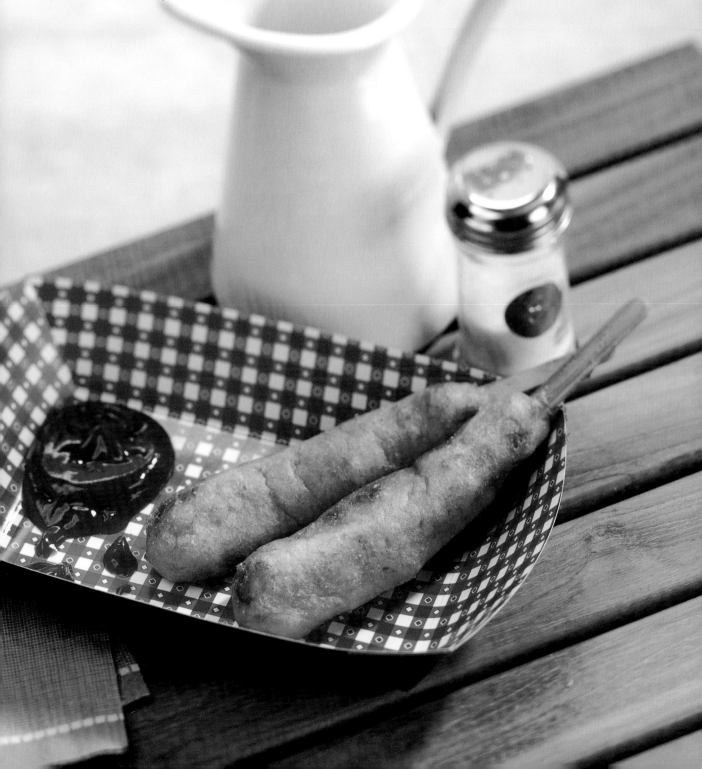

# Focaccia

## Makes 5 large or 10 small pieces

A wonderful, chewy flatbread with a Mediterranean twist. You can either spread the batter or roll it out—use sweet rice flour for dusting. The batter includes herbs and a topping of feta, olives and sun-dried tomatoes.

1/2 cup (125 mL) warm water

1 Tbsp (15 mL) active dry yeast

2 tsp (10 mL) sugar

1 1/2 cups (375 mL) tapioca starch

1 cup (250 mL) white rice flour

1/2 cup (125 mL) sweet rice flour

1/4 cup (60 mL) whey powder

2 Tbsp (30 mL) pea fibre 80

2 Tbsp (30 mL) sugar

4 tsp (20 mL) xanthan gum

1 tsp (5 mL) dough improver (see page 9)

1 tsp (5 mL) dried oregano

1 tsp (5 mL) salt

1/2 tsp (2 mL) dried thyme

1/4 tsp (1 mL) dried marjoram

1 1/4 cups (300 mL) water

4 egg whites (large), room temperature

3 Tbsp (45 mL) cooking oil

1/2 cup (125 mL) crumbled feta cheese

1/2 cup (125 mL) grated mozzarella cheese

1/2 cup (125 mL) sliced black olives

1/4 cup (60 mL) sun-dried tomatoes

2 Tbsp (30 mL) grated Parmesan cheese

Place first 3 ingredients in a small bowl. Let stand for 10 minutes until foamy.

Mix next 12 ingredients in a large bowl.

Mix next 3 ingredients in a separate bowl. Add egg white mixture and yeast mixture to flour mixture. Stir until a smooth batter is formed. Divide batter equally into 4 parts and form into oval shapes on a greased baking sheet. Smooth with a wet spatula.

Mix remaining 5 ingredients in a separate bowl. Spread over batter. Place in a warm place and cover with a damp towel. Let rise for 15 to 20 minutes until about doubled in size. Bake on middle rack of a 400°F (200°C) oven for 20 to 25 minutes until bread sounds hollow when tapped. Let stand on a wire rack to cool.

*1 large piece: 564 Calories; 20 g Total Fat (9 g Mono, 3 g Poly, 5 g Sat); 31 mg Cholesterol; 84 g Carbohydrate; 7 g Fibre; 15 g Protein; 1080 mg Sodium*

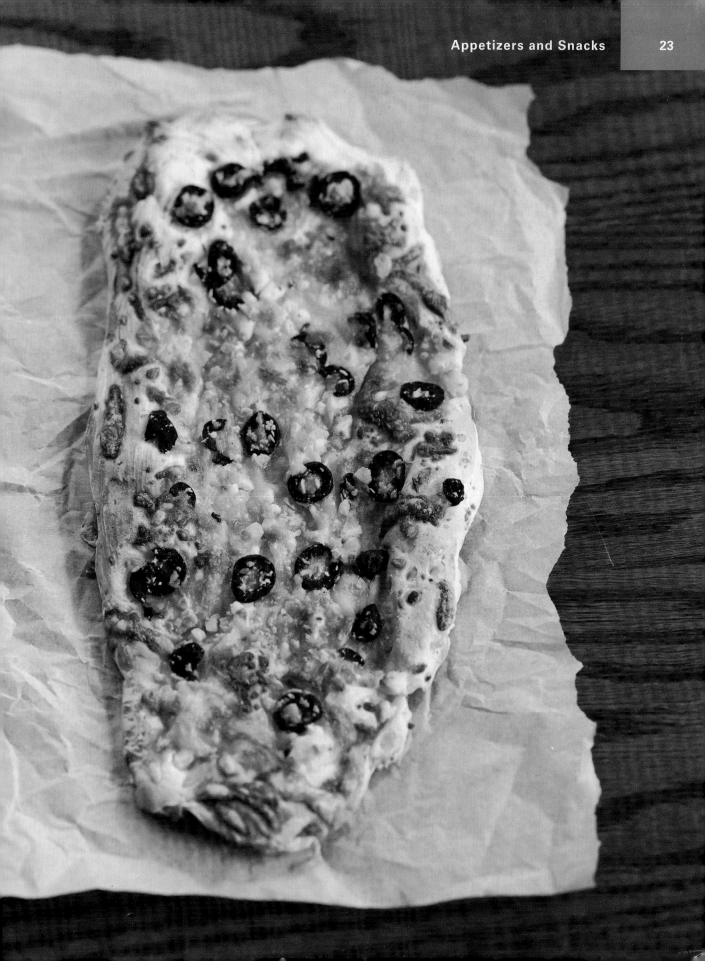

# Garlic Bread Sticks

## Makes 12 to 15

Serve these flavourful bread sticks as a side dish to a meal or as a snack between meals. I also like them simply by themselves with a nice dipping sauce such as a raspberry chipotle. These bread sticks are best fresh, but will be good for a day if stored in a plastic bag or container.

1/2 cup (125 mL) warm water

1 Tbsp (15 mL) active dry yeast

2 tsp (10 mL) sugar

3/4 cup (175 mL) tapioca starch

1/2 cup (125 mL) white rice flour

1/4 cup (60 mL) sweet rice flour

2 Tbsp (30 mL) whey powder

1 Tbsp (15 mL) pea fibre 80

1 Tbsp (15 mL) xanthan gum

1 Tbsp (15 mL) sugar

1/2 tsp (2 mL) salt

1/2 tsp (2 mL) dough improver (see page 9)

1/2 to 3/4 cup (125 to 175 mL) water

2 Tbsp (30 mL) cooking oil

2 egg whites, room temperature

olive oil, for brushing

garlic powder or garlic salt, for sprinkling

paprika powder, for sprinkling (optional)

Place first 3 ingredients in a small bowl. Let stand for 10 minutes until foamy.

Mix next 9 ingredients in a large bowl.

Mix next 3 ingredients in a separate bowl. Add egg mixture and yeast mixture to flour mixture. Stir until a smooth batter is formed. Scoop batter into a pastry bag without a tip. Pipe batter onto greased baking sheets into logs 1/4 to 1/2 inch (6 to 12 mm) thick and 6 to 10 inches (15 to 25 cm) long. Place in a warm place and cover with a damp towel. Let rise for 15 to 20 minutes until about doubled in size.

Brush the bread dough with olive oil and sprinkle with garlic powder or garlic salt. Place pans on middle rack of a 375°F (190°C) oven and bake for 20 to 25 minutes until golden brown. Remove from pan. Sprinkle with paprika before serving if desired.

*1 bread stick: 79 Calories; 2 g Total Fat (1 g Mono, 1 g Poly, 0 g Sat); 1 mg Cholesterol; 14 g Carbohydrate; 1 g Fibre; 2 g Protein; 101 mg Sodium*

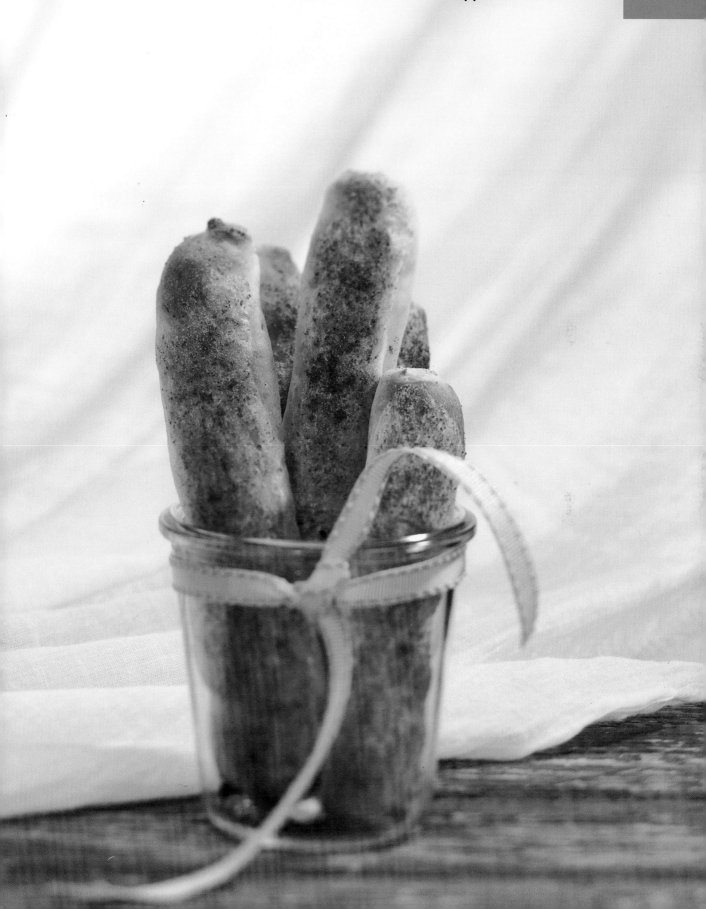

# Tortillas and Dip

## Serves 8

A nice twist that can be used in any tortilla dish and fried for chips as well. It's a little tricky to work with, but well worth the time. Add a favourite seasoning and you have a great thin flatbread for your South American–influenced supper. For the dip, you can keep the ingredients separate in individual dipping bowls or combine them into a delicious layer dip in a large glass bowl.

### Tortillas

2 cups (500 mL) masa harina

2/3 cup (150 mL) sweet rice flour

2/3 cup (150 mL) tapioca starch

1/3 cup (75 mL) pea starch

1 1/2 Tbsp (25 mL) pea fibre III

1 Tbsp (15 mL) xanthan gum

1 1/4 tsp (6 mL) guar gum

1 1/2 to 2 cups (375 to 500 mL) water

3 Tbsp (45 mL) cooking oil

### Dip

3 ripe avocados, mashed

juice from 1 lemon

1/8 tsp (0.5 mL) salt

1/8 tsp (0.5 mL) pepper

1/2 cup (125 mL) sour cream

2 Tbsp (30 mL) salsa (mild or hot, to taste)

*(continued on next page)*

**Tortillas:** Mix first 7 ingredients in a medium metal bowl.

Mix remaining 2 ingredients in a separate bowl. Add water mixture to flour mixture. Knead together or use a heavy-duty mixer with a dough hook attachment. Turn out dough onto surface lightly dusted with sweet rice flour. Divide dough into 20 balls, about 2 oz each. Press each out in a tortilla maker, or roll out each very thinly. Cook in ungreased nonstick pan on medium for 2 to 4 minutes per side until just starting to brown.

**Dip:** Combine first 6 ingredients in a medium bowl. Mix well.

Mash up beans. Add taco seasoning. Stir.

To assemble, layer ingredients in a medium glass bowl as follows:

• Avocado dip

• Bean mixture

• Cheese

• Green onions

• Tomatoes

Serve spoonfuls of dip with tortilla rounds.

*1 serving:* 578 Calories; 28 g Total Fat (12 g Mono, 4 g Poly, 7 g Sat); 21 mg Cholesterol; 73 g Carbohydrate; 16 g Fibre; 16 g Protein; 491 mg Sodium

## Tip

You can make your own gluten-free taco seasoning. Just mix 1/2 tsp (2 mL) *each* of chili powder, ground cumin and paprika with 1/4 tsp (1 mL) *each* of garlic powder and onion powder.

1 x 14 oz (398 mL) can of gluten-free refried beans

1 to 2 tsp (5 to 10 mL) gluten-free taco seasoning (see Tip)

1 cup (250 mL) grated medium Cheddar cheese

1/4 to 1/2 cup (60 to 125 mL) sliced green onions

1/2 cup (125 mL) diced tomato

# Potato Pancakes

## Makes 7

A classic in our house when we lived in Germany. Pan-fried in lard or duck fat and served with applesauce or fruit compote, this traditional recipe is best served hot.

**1 Tbsp (15 mL) gluten-free all-purpose flour (see page 9)**

**1 1/2 tsp (7 mL) salt**

**1/2 tsp (2 mL) baking powder**

**2 cups (500 mL) peeled, grated potatoes**

**2 large eggs, fork-beaten**

**2 Tbsp (30 mL) grated onion**

**2 to 4 Tbsp (30 to 60 mL) lard (or duck fat or cooking oil)**

**applesauce or fruit compote, for topping (optional)**

Mix first 3 ingredients in a small bowl.

Squeeze grated potatoes to remove excess water. Mix potatoes, eggs and onion in a medium bowl. Add flour mixture to potato mixture. Beat well.

Heat a large frying pan on high. Add 1 to 2 Tbsp (15 to 30 mL) lard. Pour batter onto frying pan, using 1/4 to 1/3 cup (60 to 75 mL) for each pancake. Spread out the batter to form flat pancakes. Cook for about 2 minutes until bubbles form on top and edges appear dry. Turn pancake over. Cook for another 2 minutes until golden. Remove to a large plate. Cover to keep warm. Repeat with remaining batter, adding more lard to frying pan if necessary to prevent sticking.

Serve pancakes hot with applesauce or fruit compote.

*1 pancake: 111 Calories; 5 g Total Fat (3 g Mono, 1 g Poly, 1 g Sat); 53 mg Cholesterol; 13 g Carbohydrate; 1 g Fibre; 3 g Protein; 543 mg Sodium*

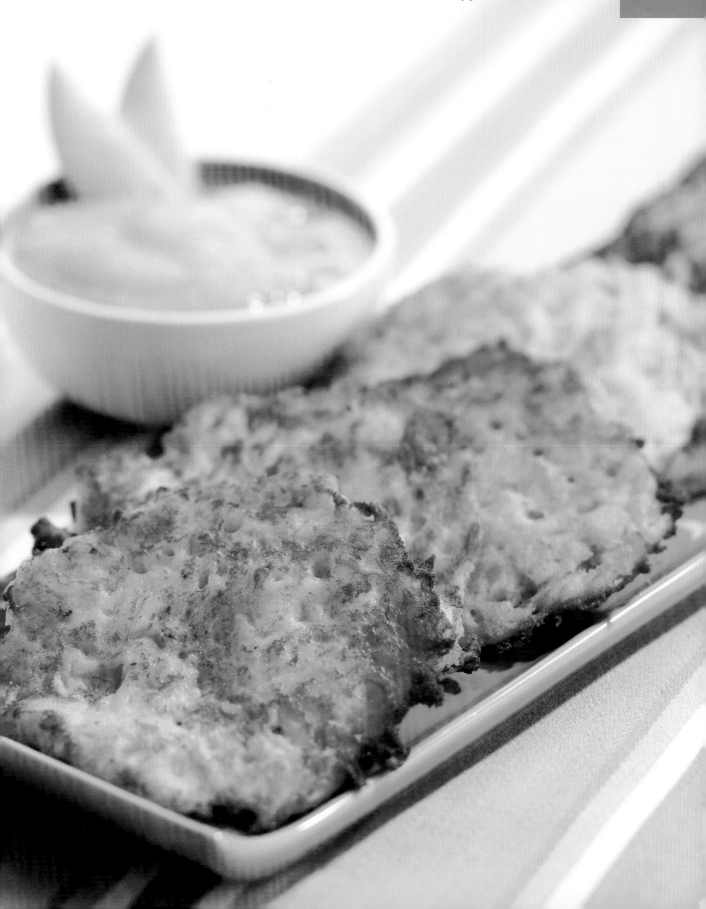

# Chris's Frittata Tarts

## Makes 12 muffin-sized frittatas

I was offered these fantastic frittata tarts for the first time by a very special person on a brilliant, sunny fall day. These are so good I had to include Chris's recipe in this book. They are excellent for breakfast but honestly are great at any time of the day. The basic recipe comes first, and you will find suggested variations below—or try your own! The frittata tarts also can be frozen to eat later.

**1 cup (250 mL) grated cheese (see chart)**

**1 cup (250 mL) crumbled precooked meat (see chart)**

**3/4 to 1 cup (175 to 250 mL) finely chopped vegetables (see chart)**

**8 large eggs**

**1/3 cup (75 mL) half-and-half cream**

**1 to 2 tsp (5 to 10 mL) seasoning (see chart)**

Preheat oven to 350°F (175°C). Grease 12 muffin cups. Mix cheese, meat and vegetables together in a medium bowl. Divide mixture evenly among muffin cups.

Whisk together eggs and cream in a separate medium bowl. Pour into each cup until cheese mixture is just covered. Sprinkle with seasoning. Bake in preheated oven for 20 to 25 minutes until knife inserted in centre of tart comes out clean.

*1 Lorraine tart:* 132 Calories; 10 g Total Fat (4 g Mono, 1 g Poly, 4 g Sat); 144 mg Cholesterol; 1 g Carbohydrate; 0 g Fibre; 10 g Protein; 143 mg Sodium

| Variations | Cheese | Meat | Vegetable | Seasoning |
|---|---|---|---|---|
| Lorraine | Gruyère | Bacon | Green onion | Dry mustard |
| Reuben | Swiss | Corn beef | 3/4 cup (175 mL) well-drained sauerkraut 1/4 cup (60 mL) green pepper | Mixed herbs |
| Sausage & Spinach | Cheddar | Pork sausage | 3/4 cup (175 mL) frozen spinach, thawed and well-drained | Caraway seed |
| Ham | Cheddar | Ham | 3/4 cup (175 mL) cooked broccoli or asparagus 1/4 cup (60 mL) green pepper | Basil |
| Italian | Mozzarella | Salami or pepperoni | 1/2 cup (125 mL) mushrooms 1/4 cup (60 mL) red pepper | Oregano |
| Greek (vegetarian) | Feta | N/A | 1/2 cup (125 mL) black olives 1/2 cup (125 mL) green pepper 1/2 cup (125 mL) red onion 1/2 cup (125 mL) tomatoes | Dill |

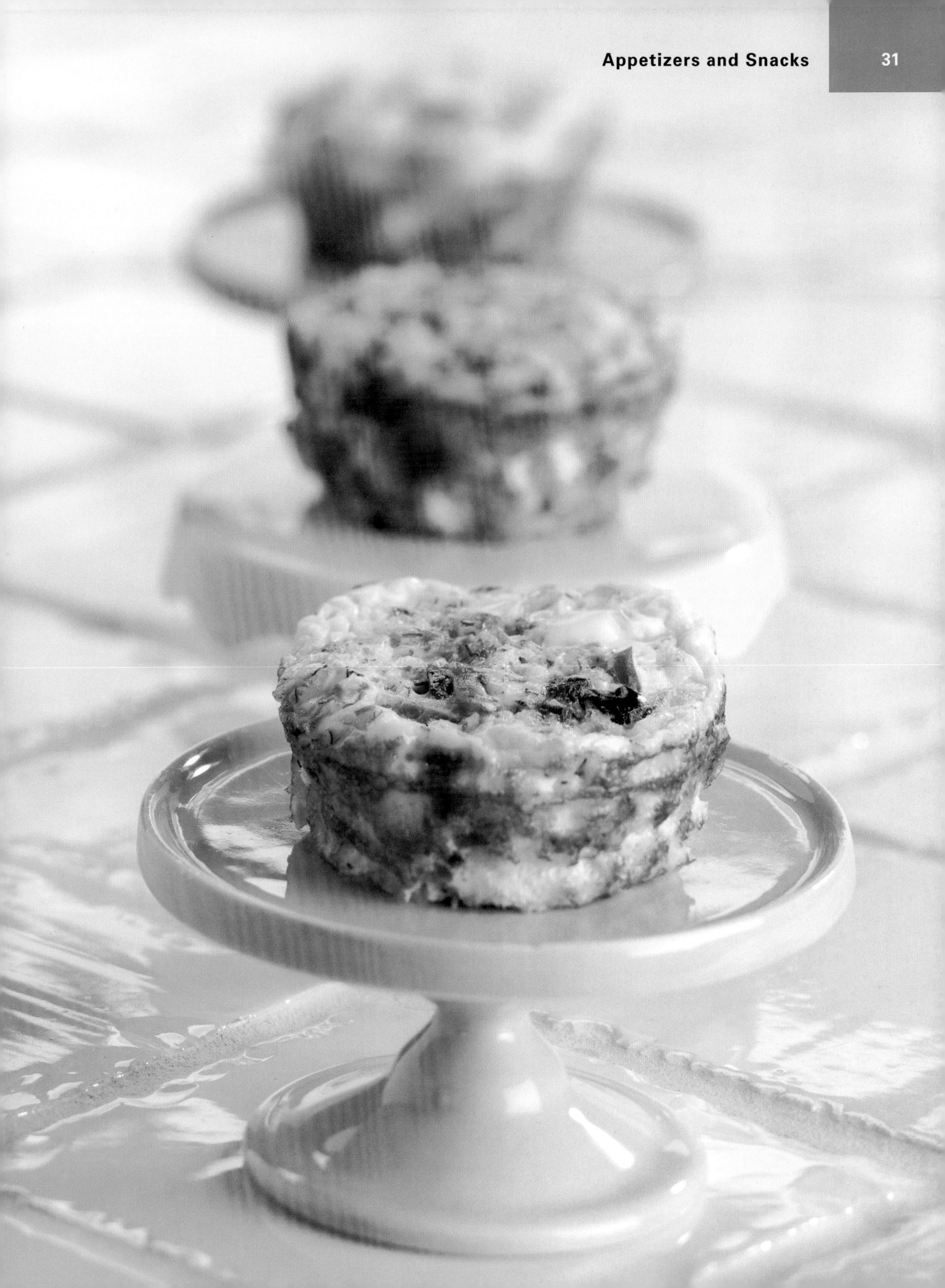

# Classic Chicken Soup

## Makes 12 cups

A tasty, nutritious small meal option that could also be a between-meals snack. This classic chicken stock uses the traditional German vegetable trio of celery root, leek and carrot as part of the ingredients. A good quality chicken will offer the best results, and I always make sure to get one that includes the organs and neck. Use the broth by itself in place of prepared chicken broth in other recipes, or as a gravy and sauce base. When you make this broth at home, you can be sure that it's gluten-free.

**8 to 12 cups (2 to 3 L) water**

**5 to 6 lb (2.3 to 2.7 kg) whole chicken (with neck and organs)**

**1 Tbsp (15 mL) salt**

**2 large carrots, cut into 1/2 inch (12 mm) slices**

**1 1/2 to 2 leek stalks (white part only), cut into 1/2 inch (12 mm) slices**

**1 medium celery root, peeled and cut into 1/2 inch (12 mm) slices**

**1 medium onion, halved**

**1/2 cup (125 mL) cooked white rice**

**salt and pepper, to taste**

**2 Tbsp (30 mL) fresh parsley**

Bring water to a boil in a large pot. Rinse chicken, neck and organs under cold running water, then place chicken, neck and organs in boiling water. Add salt. Heat until hot, but not boiling. Skim and discard any fat from surface of liquid.

Add next 4 ingredients. Reduce heat to low. Simmer, uncovered, for 1 1/2 to 2 hours. Remove from heat. Remove chicken and bones to cutting board using a slotted spoon. Strain stock through a sieve into a separate large pot. Discard solids.

This stock can be made into a soup or used as a broth in other recipes. It will store, covered, in the refrigerator for 3 to 4 days, or put in smaller freezer-safe containers and stored in the freezer. To make soup, remove chicken meat from bones. Discard bones and skin. Chop chicken. Add chopped chicken and rice to stock. Add salt and pepper to taste. Garnish with fresh parsley.

*1 serving:* 200 Calories; 2 g Total Fat (1 g Mono, 0 g Poly, 1 g Sat); 99 mg Cholesterol; 3 g Carbohydrate; 0 g Fibre; 40 g Protein; 982 mg Sodium

To avoid crying when cutting onions, keep a bit of water in your mouth.

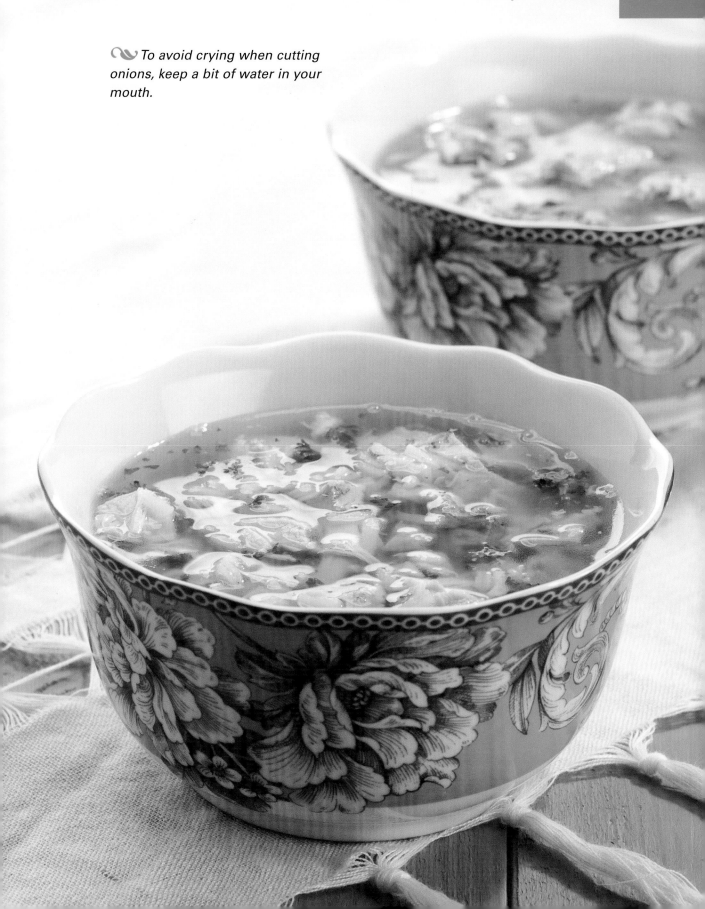

# Classic Beef Stock

## Makes 12 cups

A potent tasty broth—well worth the extra effort. This classic beef stock uses beef bones with celery, carrots, onions and herbs in a two-step process to make a strong reduction that will serve as a wonderful base for many recipes. It's also tasty served hot in a mug on its own.

**6 lbs (2.7 kg) fresh beef bones**

**4 to 5 celery stalks, halved lengthwise and cut into 1/2 inch (12 mm) slices**

**2 large carrots, cut into 1/2 inch (12 mm) slices**

**2 medium tomatoes, halved**

**1 large onion, halved**

**2 Tbsp (30 mL) tomato paste**

**2 Tbsp (30 mL) rice vinegar**

**1 Tbsp (15 mL) fancy (mild) molasses**

**1 sprig of fresh thyme**

**1/2 sprig of fresh rosemary**

**1 bay leaf**

Preheat oven to 400°F (200°C). Place beef bones and next 4 ingredients in a large roasting pan. Bake for 20 to 30 minutes until vegetables are golden brown and caramelized. Add a little water to roasting pan, stirring and scraping any brown bits from bottom of pan.

Transfer bones, vegetables and brown bits to a large pot. Add cold water until about 1 inch (2.5 cm) above bones. Add remaining 6 ingredients. Bring to a rolling boil on high. Reduce heat to medium-low. Simmer, covered, for 4 hours. Strain stock through a sieve into a separate large pot. Discard solids. Simmer, uncovered, for 35 to 50 minutes until a third of liquid is evaporated. It will store, covered, in the refrigerator for 3 to 4 days, or put in smaller freezer-safe containers and store in the freezer.

*1 pot of stock:* 113 Calories; 0 g Total Fat (0 g Mono, 0 g Poly, 0 g Sat); 0 mg Cholesterol; 28 g Carbohydrate; 3 g Fibre; 1 g Protein; 121 mg Sodium

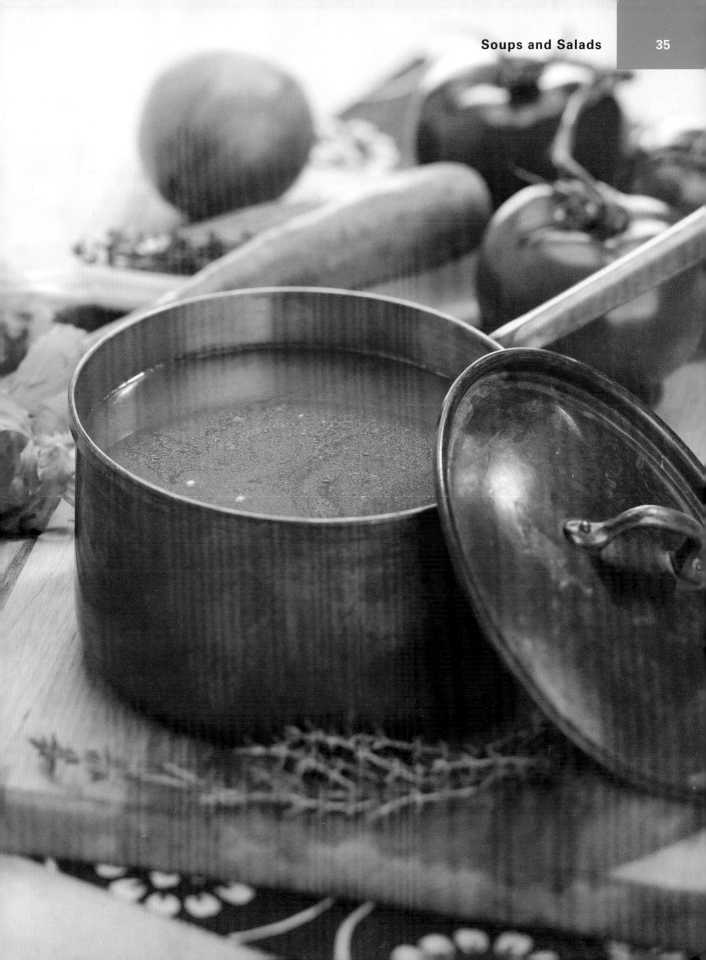

# Clam Chowder

## Makes 10 1/2 cups

Good on any day, this clam chowder follows the traditional thick and creamy concept of New England's classic. Adjust the consistency by adding more gluten-free flour if desired.

1 1/2 cups (375 mL) water

6 large potatoes, unpeeled and cubed

3 medium carrots, chopped

2 celery stalks, thinly sliced

1 1/2 cups (375 mL) chopped onion

reserved clam juice (see clams below)

1 1/2 to 2 Tbsp (25 to 30 mL) gluten-free all-purpose flour (see page 9)

6 to 7 bacon slices, cooked crisp and crumbled

4 1/2 cups (1.1 L) half-and-half cream

3 x 5 oz (142 g) cans of whole baby clams, chopped, and juice reserved

1 1/2 tsp (7 mL) salt

1/4 tsp (1 mL) pepper

paprika, for garnish

butter (optional)

Combine first 6 ingredients in a large pot. Bring to a boil on high. Reduce heat to medium-low and simmer, covered, for about 15 minutes until vegetables are soft.

Add flour. Stir. Add remaining 5 ingredients. Simmer, uncovered, for 10 to 12 minutes until slightly thickened.

Serve hot in individual bowls. Sprinkle with paprika. If desired, add a dab of butter to each bowl.

*1 cup:* 365 Calories; 14 g Total Fat (4 g Mono, 1 g Poly, 7 g Sat); 67 mg Cholesterol; 47 g Carbohydrate; 4 g Fibre; 17 g Protein; 737 mg Sodium

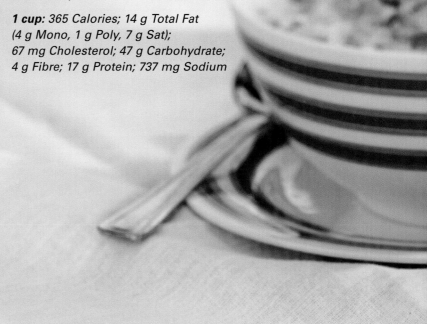

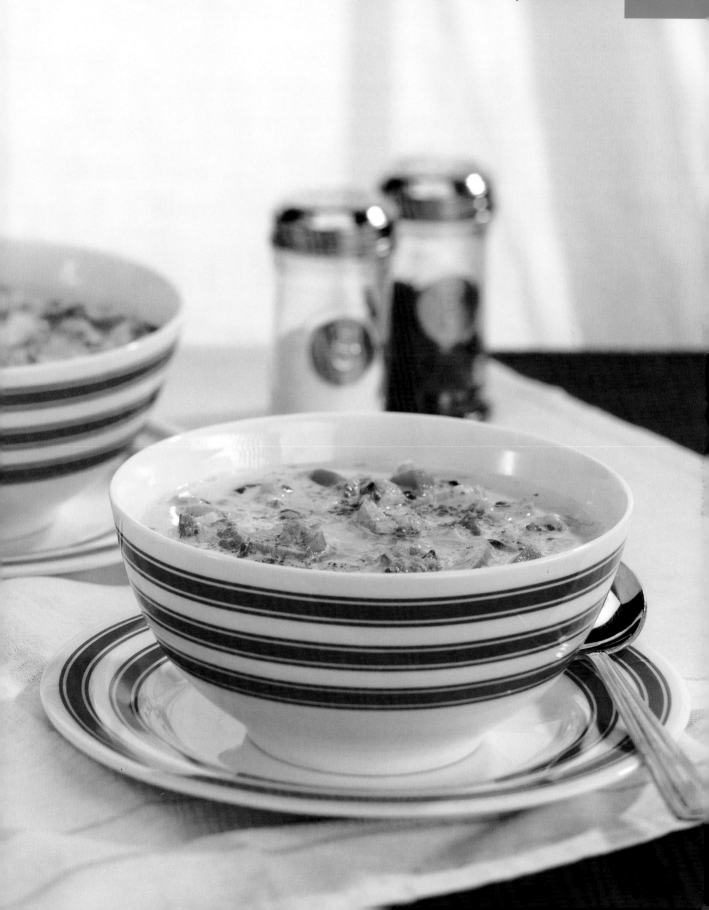

# Minestrone

## Makes 10 cups

A traditional soup from the Mediterranean area that's served over pasta with steaming hot French garlic toast. This version is prepared simply with the use of a slow cooker.

1 tsp (5 mL) canola oil

1 x 19 oz (540 mL) can of red kidney (or mixed) beans, rinsed and drained

1 x 14 oz (398 mL) can of diced tomatoes (with juice)

4 cups (1 L) chicken (or vegetable) broth

3 large carrots, thinly sliced

2 celery stalks, thinly sliced

1 large onion, finely chopped

2 Tbsp (30 mL) tomato paste

2 tsp (10 mL) crushed garlic

2 tsp (10 mL) Italian seasoning

1/4 cup (60 mL) grated Parmesan cheese

1/4 cup (60 mL) pesto

1/8 tsp (0.5 mL) pepper

1 loaf gluten-free French bread (see page 9)

2 tsp (10 mL) butter

1 tsp (5 mL) garlic powder

1/2 tsp (2 mL) parsley flakes

2 cups (500 mL) gluten-free corn elbow macaroni

Add first 13 ingredients to slow cooker. Stir. Cook, covered, on Low for 8 hours or on High for 4 to 5 hours.

Preheat oven to 350°F (175°C). Slice French bread loaf in half lengthwise. Spread butter on each side. Sprinkle with garlic powder and parsley. Place, buttered side up, on a baking sheet. Bake for 12 to 15 minutes until edges are golden brown. Let stand until cool enough to handle. Cut into 1-inch (2.5 cm) slices.

Cook pasta according to package directions for *al dente*. Drain. Divide pasta among individual serving bowls. Pour minestrone over pasta. Serve with garlic bread.

*1 serving (with bread): 657 Calories; 11 g Total Fat (1 g Mono, 0 g Poly, 3 g Sat); 15 mg Cholesterol; 123 g Carbohydrate; 19 g Fibre; 20 g Protein; 1132 mg Sodium*

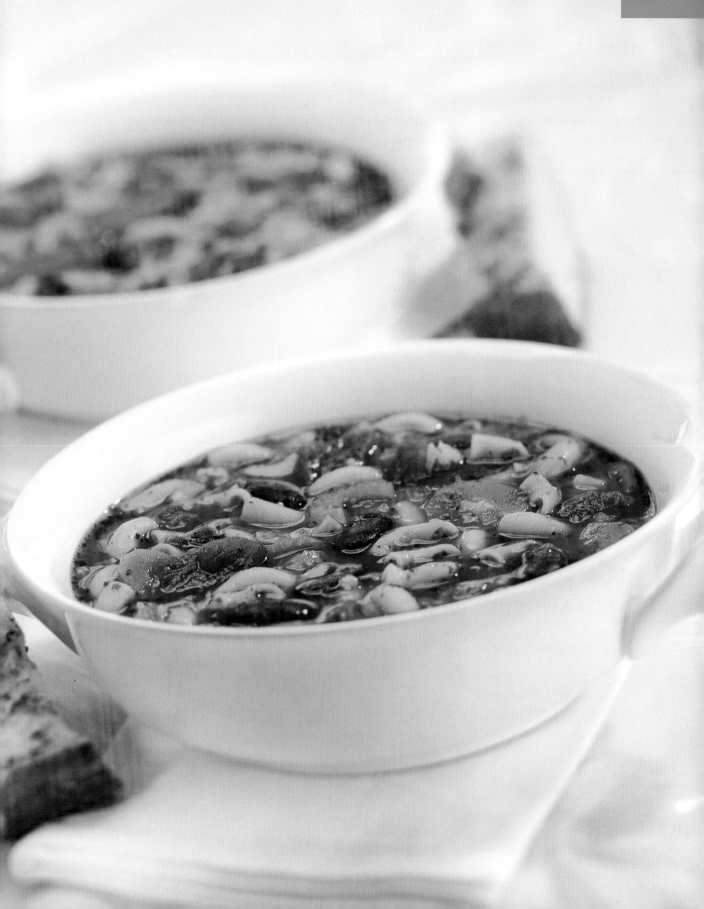

# Wild Mushroom Soup

## Makes 10 cups

A creamy wild mushroom soup with a distinct flavour. This soup is enjoyable by itself or as a base for other recipes.

**6 large potatoes, unpeeled and chopped**

**3 medium carrots, chopped**

**2 celery stalks, thinly sliced**

**2 cups (500 mL) dried wild mushrooms, finely chopped**

**1 1/2 cups (375 mL) chopped onion**

**1 1/2 cups (375 mL) water**

**1 1/2 to 2 Tbsp (25 to 30 mL) gluten-free all-purpose flour (see page 9)**

**4 1/2 cups (1.1 L) half-and-half cream**

**2 tsp (10 mL) gluten-free soy sauce**

**1 1/2 tsp (7 mL) salt**

**1/4 tsp (1 mL) pepper**

**parsley, for garnish**

Combine first 6 ingredients in a large pot. Bring to a boil on high. Reduce heat to medium-low and simmer, covered, for about 15 minutes until vegetables are soft.

Add flour. Stir. Add remaining 4 ingredients. Simmer, uncovered, for 10 to 12 minutes until slightly thickened.

Serve hot in individual bowls. Sprinkle with parsley.

*1 cup:* 456 Calories; 12 g Total Fat (3 g Mono, 1 g Poly, 7 g Sat); 34 mg Cholesterol; 83 g Carbohydrate; 10 g Fibre; 13 g Protein; 493 mg Sodium

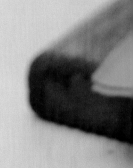

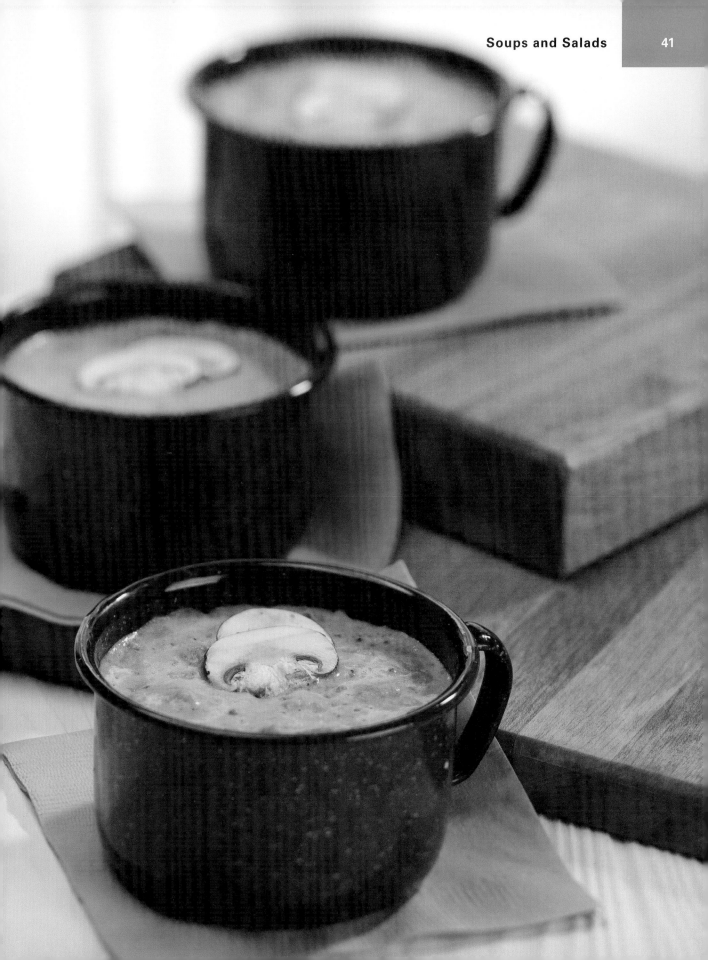

# Quinoa Salad

## Serves 6

You can make this high-protein, gluten-free grain salad as a side dish, but it also can be served as a main dish on its own. Quinoa is prepared similarly to rice, but the cooking time is much shorter.

**2 cups (500 mL) quinoa, rinsed and drained**

**4 to 5 cups (1 to 1.25 L) chicken broth**

Combine quinoa and chicken broth in a large pot. Bring to a boil on medium-high. Boil gently, uncovered, for about 10 minutes. Remove from heat. Cover to keep warm.

**1 cup (250 mL) broccoli florets**

Cook broccoli in boiling salted water or a steamer for 5 minutes until tender-crisp. Drain. Set aside to cool.

**1 Tbsp (15 mL) cooking oil**

**2 x 4 to 6 oz (113 to 170 g) boneless, skinless chicken breast halves**

**1 Tbsp (15 mL) gluten-free tamari sauce**

Heat cooking oil in a frying pan on medium. Add chicken and tamari sauce. Cook for 4 to 5 minutes per side, turning chicken breasts every 2 minutes, until no longer pink inside. Remove from heat. Set aside and cool.

Combine next 6 ingredients in a small bowl.

**1/2 cup (125 mL) lemon juice**

**1/3 cup (75 mL) olive oil**

**1 garlic clove, minced**

**1 Tbsp (15 mL) Dijon mustard**

**1/4 tsp (1 mL) salt**

**1/4 tsp (1 mL) pepper**

Place remaining 4 ingredients in a large bowl. Cut cooled broccoli and chicken into small pieces and add to large bowl. Add olive oil mixture and stir well. Add quinoa 1/2 cup (125 mL) at a time, stirring well after each addition. Let stand at room temperature for 30 to 60 minutes before serving.

*1 serving:* 424 Calories; 19 g Total Fat (12 g Mono, 3 g Poly, 2 g Sat); 17 mg Cholesterol; 51 g Carbohydrate; 5 g Fibre; 16 g Protein; 765 mg Sodium

**2 medium tomatoes, diced**

**1 large English cucumber, diced**

**1 large red pepper, diced**

**1 small red onion, diced**

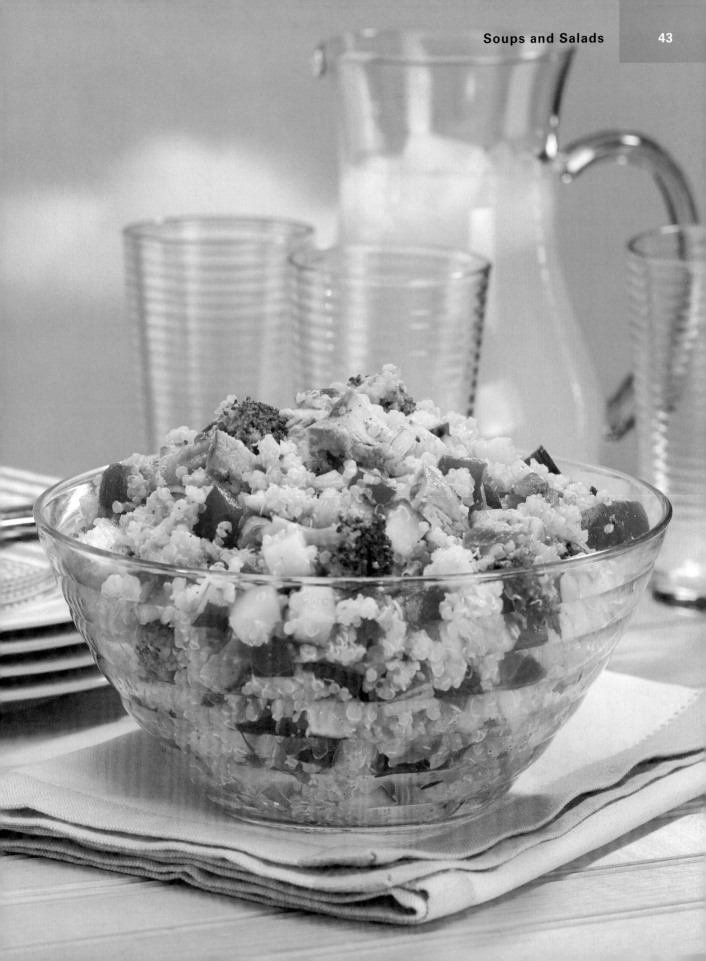

# Caesar Salad

## Serves 6 to 8

A classic! This romaine lettuce–based meal with distinct creamy dressing and gluten-free croutons satisfies as a meal or side dish. This version uses a rich yogurt instead of the traditional raw egg ingredients. If you're comfortable that you have a safe source of eggs, you can use 2 egg yolks in place of the Greek yogurt.

**8 anchovies, mashed, or 2 to 3 Tbsp (30 to 45 mL) anchovy paste**

**juice from 1 to 1 1/2 lemons**

**1/2 cup (125 mL) grated Parmesan cheese**

**1/2 to 3/4 cup (125 to 175 mL) olive oil**

**1/4 to 1/3 cup (60 to 75 mL) red wine vinegar**

**1/4 cup (60 mL) plain Greek yogurt**

**2 Tbsp (30 mL) Dijon mustard**

**2 Tbsp (30 mL) minced garlic**

**1/8 tsp (0.5 mL) apple cider vinegar**

**1/8 tsp (0.5 mL) gluten-free tamari sauce**

**1/8 tsp (0.5 mL) pepper**

**dash of garlic powder**

**2 heads of romaine lettuce, cut or torn**

**1 1/2 to 2 cups (375 to 500 mL) gluten-free croutons**

Process first 12 ingredients together in a blender or food processor until smooth.

Toss lettuce with dressing in an extra large bowl. Add croutons. Toss lightly.

*1 serving: 421 Calories; 23 g Total Fat (14 g Mono, 2 g Poly, 5 g Sat); 20 mg Cholesterol; 45 g Carbohydrate; 7 g Fibre; 11 g Protein; 899 mg Sodium*

*To make gluten-free croutons, I cut gluten-free French bread (see page 9) into 3/4 inch (2 mm) cubes. Toss the bread cubes with 1/4 cup (60 mL) olive oil and a sprinkle of salt and pepper. Bake on an ungreased baking sheet with sides in a 375ºF (190ºC) oven for 6 to 10 minutes until golden.*

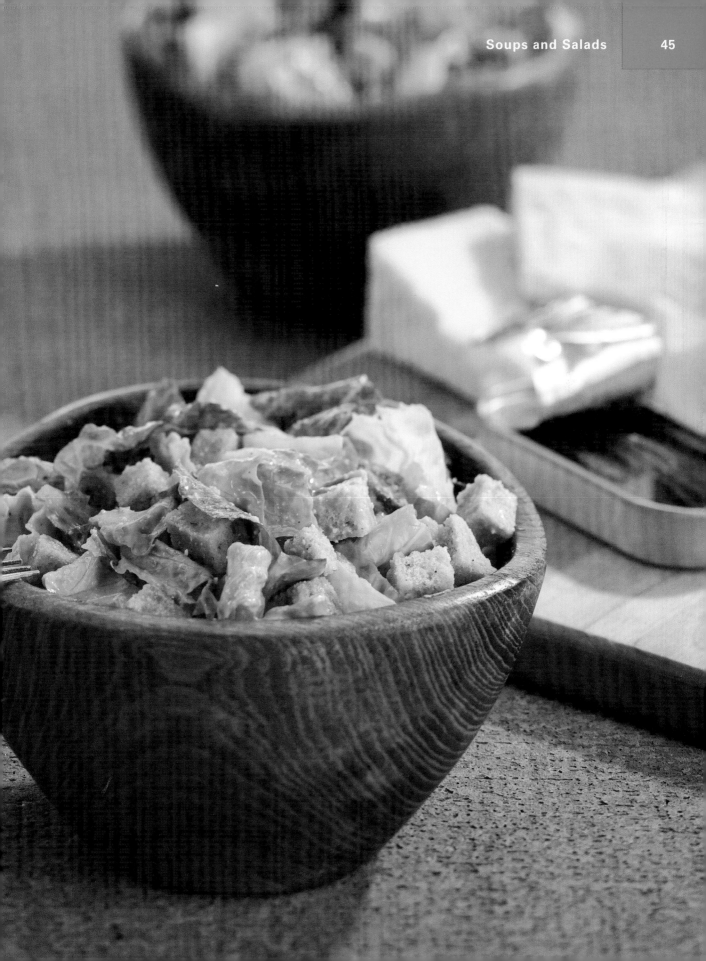

# Waldorf Salad

## Serves 6 to 8

First known to be served in the famous Waldorf–Astoria hotel, this salad is welcome at potlucks anytime and enjoyed by even the pickiest eaters.

**3 large apples (such as Gala or McIntosh), cut into 3/4 inch (2 cm) pieces**

**3 celery stalks, thinly sliced**

**1 cup (250 mL) seedless green grapes, halved**

**3/4 cup (175 mL) walnut pieces**

**1/3 to 1/2 cup (75 to 125 mL) mayonnaise**

**1/3 to 1/2 cup (75 to 125 mL) plain yogurt**

**3 Tbsp (45 mL) lemon juice**

**1 medium head of butter lettuce**

Place first 3 ingredients in a large bowl.

Brown walnut pieces in a frying pan for 3 to 4 minutes, stirring occasionally, until slightly toasted. Add to the bowl containing the fruit and celery.

Combine next 3 ingredients in a small bowl until well mixed. Add to fruit and celery. Toss well. Chill, covered, in refrigerator for 1 hour.

Serve on butter lettuce leaves.

*1 serving: 275 Calories; 20 g Total Fat (1 g Mono, 7 g Poly, 3 g Sat); 6 mg Cholesterol; 24 g Carbohydrate; 4 g Fibre; 4 g Protein; 94 mg Sodium*

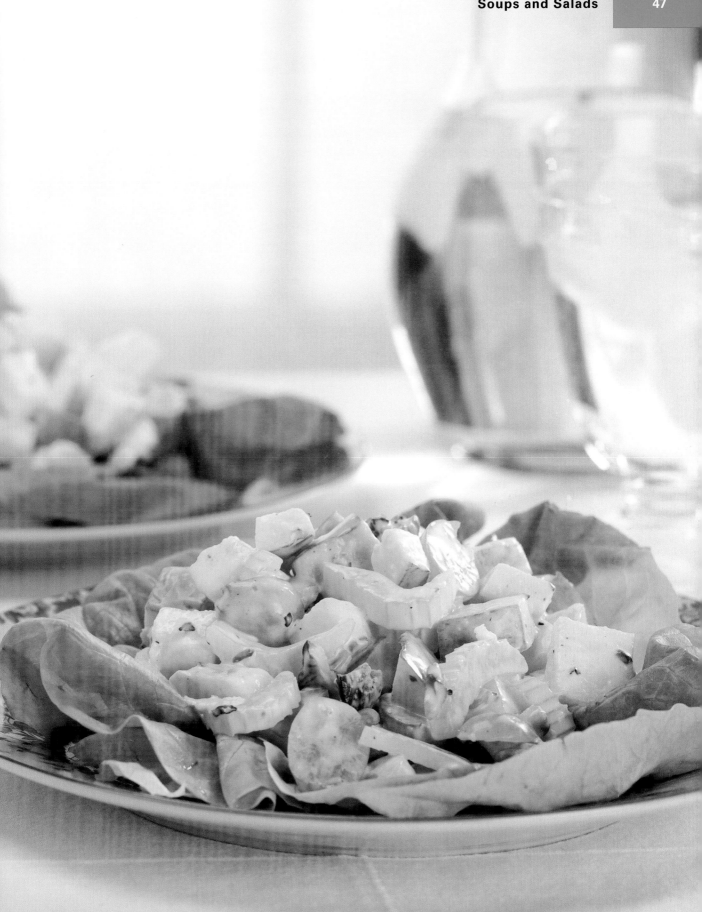

# Tuna Pasta Salad

## Serves 6 to 8

A quick satisfying meal in itself, this tasty combination of gluten-free pasta and protein rich tuna, seasoned with apple cider vinegar, lemons and mustard, can be enjoyed both warm and cold.

| | |
|---|---|
| 2 to 3 cups (500 to 750 mL) gluten-free corn pasta shells | Cook pasta according to package directions to *al dente*. Drain. Transfer to a large bowl. |

2 large carrots, thinly sliced

2 celery stalks, thinly sliced

3/4 cup (175 mL) fresh (or frozen, thawed) peas

1/4 to 1/2 cup (60 to 125 mL) sliced dill pickles

1 small red onion, finely diced

Add next 5 ingredients. Break tuna into smaller pieces and add. Toss the mixture gently.

2 x 6 oz (170 g) cans of solid white tuna in water, drained

Whisk remaining 9 ingredients in a small bowl until combined. Add to pasta. Toss. Chill, covered, in refrigerator for 5 to 8 hours before serving.

1/2 to 3/4 cup (125 to 175 mL) olive oil

1/4 to 1/3 cup (60 to 75 mL) white wine vinegar

1/4 cup (60 mL) mayonnaise

juice from 1 to 1 1/2 medium lemons

1 tsp (5 mL) Dijon mustard

1 tsp (5 mL) minced garlic

1/8 tsp (0.5 mL) apple cider vinegar

1/2 tsp (2 mL) salt

1/8 tsp (0.5 mL) pepper

*1 serving:* 470 Calories; 29 g Total Fat (14 g Mono, 3 g Poly, 4 g Sat); 27 mg Cholesterol; 37 g Carbohydrate; 5 g Fibre; 18 g Protein; 595 mg Sodium

**Variation:** Try sweet pickles instead of dill pickles.

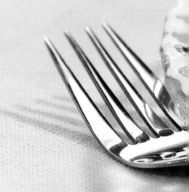

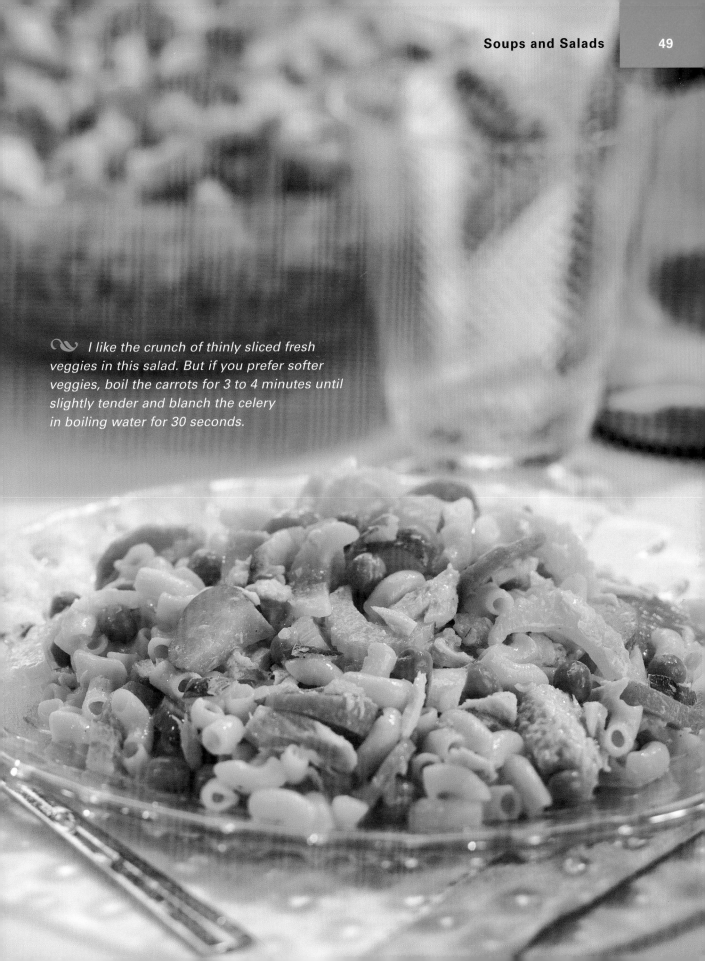

*I like the crunch of thinly sliced fresh veggies in this salad. But if you prefer softer veggies, boil the carrots for 3 to 4 minutes until slightly tender and blanch the celery in boiling water for 30 seconds.*

# Beef Stew

## Serves 6 to 8

Simmered in a slow cooker, this hearty, strong-flavoured stew is an easy one-bowl meal that warms you even on the coldest nights. Serve the stew by itself or with a slice of gluten-free French bread (see page 9).

2 Tbsp (30 mL) cooking oil

3 lbs (1.4 kg) stewing beef, cubed

2 tsp (10 mL) gluten-free teriyaki sauce (see page 156)

1 tsp (5 mL) gluten-free soy sauce

3 celery stalks, thinly sliced

3 medium carrots, thinly sliced

1 large onion, diced

1 Tbsp (15 mL) fancy (mild) molasses

1 Tbsp (15 mL) vinegar

1 x 28 oz (796 ml) can of diced tomatoes

3 large potatoes, cut into 1/2 inch (12 mm) cubes

1 cup (250 mL) beef broth

1/4 tsp (1 mL) salt

1/8 tsp (0.5 mL) pepper

1 lb (454 g) frozen French-style green beans

1/3 cup (75 mL) cold water (optional)

3 Tbsp (45 mL) cornstarch (optional)

Heat cooking oil in a large frying pan on medium. Add next 3 ingredients. Heat and stir for 2 to 3 minutes until beef is browned. Place in a large slow cooker.

Add next 10 ingredients to slow cooker. Stir. Cook, covered, on Low for 7 to 8 hours or on High for 4 to 5 hours.

Add green beans. Cook on Low for 1 hour or on High for 15 to 20 minutes.

If a thicker stew is desired, stir water into cornstarch until smooth. Add to slow cooker. Stir. Cover. Cook on High for 15 to 20 minutes.

*1 serving:* 613 Calories; 21 g Total Fat (8 g Mono, 3 g Poly, 6 g Sat); 111 mg Cholesterol; 47 g Carbohydrate; 6 g Fibre; 57 g Protein; 733 mg Sodium

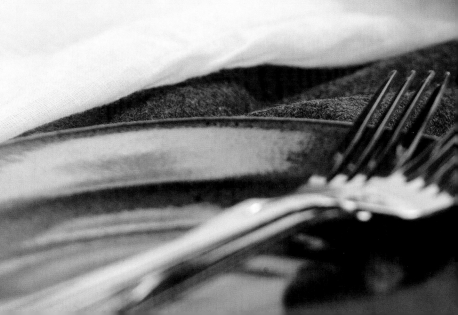

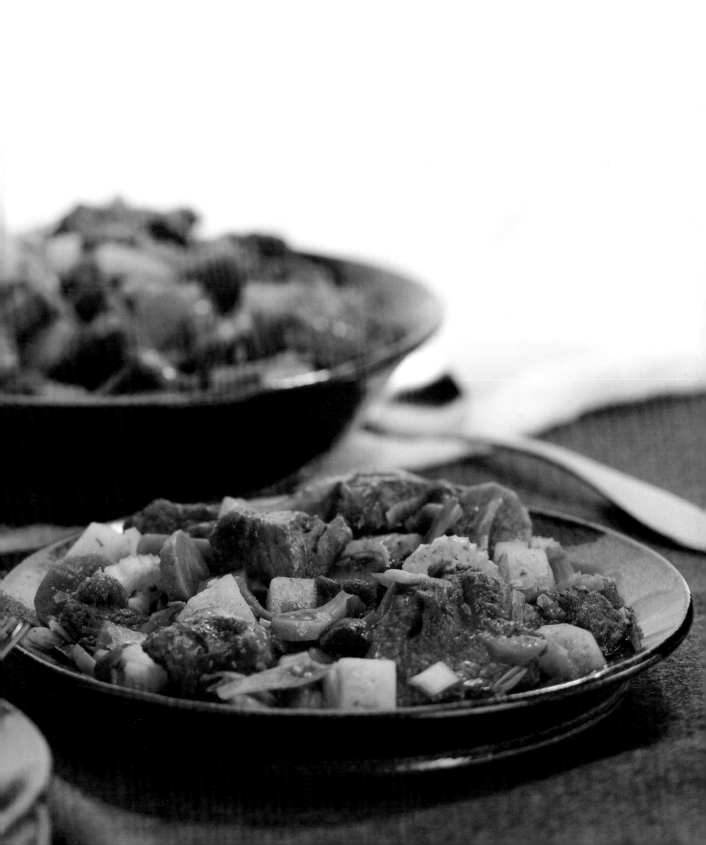

# Beef Goulash

## Serves 6

The subtle spiciness in this rich meaty dish is perfect for any cool day. A sure winner served with rolls or over Spaetzle (see page 142).

**6 bacon slices, chopped**

**4 medium onions, finely chopped**

Cook bacon in a Dutch oven until browned. Transfer with slotted spoon to paper towel–lined bowl to drain. Add onion to hot bacon drippings. Cook for about 5 minutes until softened. Transfer with slotted spoon to bowl.

**2 lb (900 g) beef pot roast, cut into 1 1/2 inch (4 cm) cubes**

**1 medium green pepper, diced**

Add beef to Dutch oven. Cook for 5 to 8 minutes, stirring occasionally, until browned on all sides. Add next 4 ingredients, as well as cooked bacon and onion.

**1 1/2 Tbsp (25 mL) Hungarian paprika**

**2 tsp (10 mL) salt**

**1/4 tsp (1 mL) pepper**

**1 cup (250 mL) dry white wine**

**2 3/4 cups (675 mL) beef broth**

Slowly add wine and beef stock, stirring. Bring to a boil. Reduce heat to low. Simmer, covered, for 2 1/2 hours.

**3/4 cup (175 mL) water**

**4 to 6 Tbsp (60 to 90 mL) gluten-free all-purpose flour (see page 9)**

Stir water into flour until smooth. Add to goulash in portions, stirring, adding only enough flour mixture to reach desired consistency. Bring to a boil, constantly stirring. Remove from heat.

**2 Tbsp (30 mL) butter**

**2 Tbsp (30 mL) water**

**1 tsp (5 mL) Hungarian paprika**

Melt butter in a small saucepan. Add water and paprika, stirring constantly until smooth. Pour sauce over goulash. Serve hot.

*1 serving: 702 Calories; 40 g Total Fat (19 g Mono, 3 g Poly, 18 g Sat); 147 mg Cholesterol; 14 g Carbohydrate; 2 g Fibre; 54 g Protein; 1451 mg Sodium*

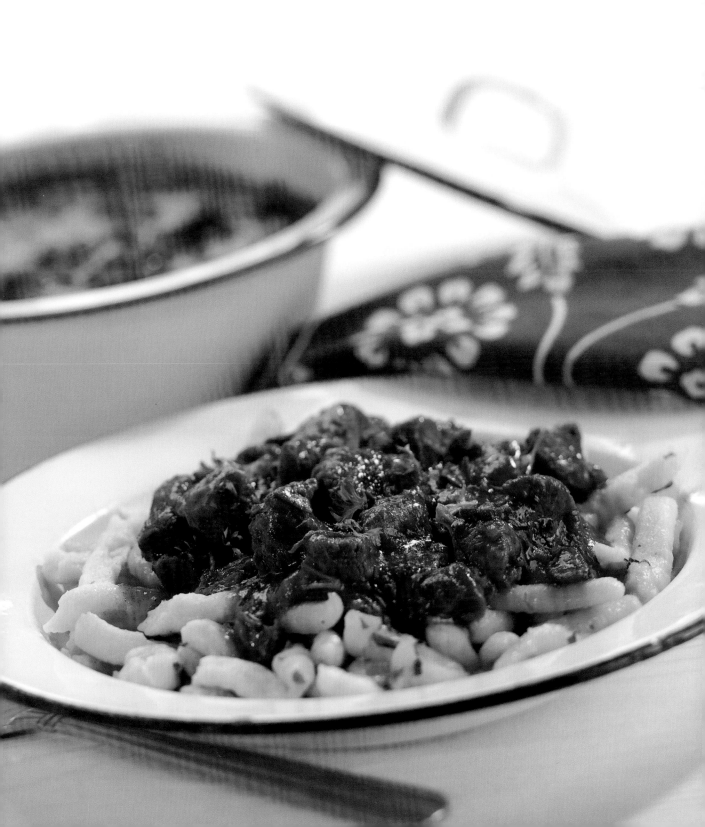

# Beef Stroganoff

## Serves 6 to 8

This tasty dish combines tender strips of sirloin, fragrant herbs and seasonings with mushrooms in a sour-cream base. Sometimes I add about 1 pound (454 grams) of green beans at the same time as the mushrooms. Serve this dish over rice.

3/4 cup (175 mL) butter

3 lb (1.4 kg) beef sirloin roast, trimmed of fat, cut into 2 x 1/2 inch (5 x 1.2 cm) strips

1 1/2 tsp (7 mL) salt

1/4 tsp (1 mL) pepper

1/4 tsp (1 mL) paprika

1/4 tsp (1 mL) dried thyme

1/2 tsp (2 mL) gluten-free steak seasoning

3/4 cup (175 mL) gluten-free all-purpose flour (see page 9)

3/4 cup (175 mL) finely chopped onions

3 cups (750 mL) beef broth

3/4 lb (340 g) fresh small white mushrooms

1 1/2 cup (375 mL) sour cream

1/3 cup (75 mL) tomato paste

1 1/2 tsp (7 mL) gluten-free teriyaki sauce (see page 156)

Melt butter in a large frying pan on medium. Add beef. Cook for 3 to 4 minutes until browned.

Add next 5 ingredients. Stir.

Push beef to one side of pan. While stirring juices on other side, add flour. Heat and stir for 1 minute. Add onions and stir mixture together. Cook for 2 minutes until onions are softened.

Gradually add beef broth. Reduce heat to low. Simmer, covered, for about 50 minutes until beef is tender.

Add mushrooms. Stir. Cook for 7 minutes. Add sour cream, tomato paste and teriyaki sauce. Cook, stirring, for 3 minutes. Remove from heat. Let sit for 5 minutes before serving over rice.

*1 serving: 848 Calories; 61 g Total Fat (20 g Mono, 2 g Poly, 32 g Sat); 179 mg Cholesterol; 21 g Carbohydrate; 3 g Fibre; 54 g Protein; 1475 mg Sodium*

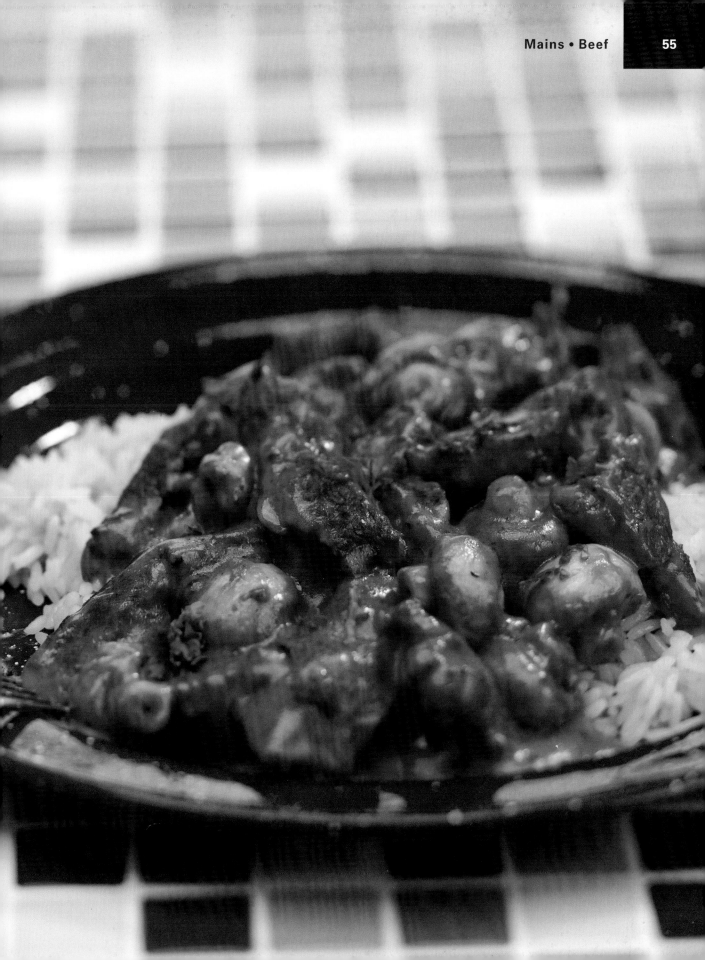

# Beef Wellington Supreme

## Serves 8

A delicious meat dish wrapped in a tender pastry—save this wonderful dinner entrée for a special occasion. It is worth the extra time and effort and will be a hit with any slow-food lover. Consider preparing the three main parts (beef tenderloin, pastry dough and ground meat) the day before. Serve with Brussels sprouts and parsley-sprinkled potatoes.

## Beef Tenderloin

**6 lb (2.7 kg) beef tenderloin roast, trimmed of fat**

**1 garlic clove, halved**

**1/4 to 1/2 tsp (1 to 2 mL) salt**

**1/4 to 1/2 tsp (1 to 2 mL) pepper**

**4 pieces suet, to cover roast (see Tip, below)**

## Ground Meat

**1/4 cup (60 mL) butter**

**1/2 cup (125 mL) finely chopped hazelnuts (filberts)**

**1/4 cup (60 mL) finely chopped onion**

**1/4 cup (60 mL) cognac**

**1/4 lb (113 g) chopped fresh white mushrooms**

**1/4 cup (60 mL) whipping cream**

**1 large egg, fork-beaten**

**1 tsp (5 mL) salt**

**1/4 tsp (1 mL) dried basil**

**1/4 tsp (1 mL) crushed dried rosemary**

**1/4 tsp (1 mL) dried thyme**

**1/8 tsp (0.5 mL) pepper**

**1/8 tsp (0.5 mL) ground allspice**

*(continued on next page)*

**Beef Tenderloin:** Preheat oven to 425°F (220°C). Rub beef with cut sides of garlic clove. Place in shallow roasting pan. Sprinkle with salt and pepper. Cover with suet. Cook in oven for about 1 hour until meat thermometer inserted in thickest part of roast reads 160°F (71°C) for medium or until desired doneness. When slightly cooled, remove suet. Cover the roast and chill for at least 1 1/2 hours.

**Ground Meat:** Heat butter in a medium saucepan on medium. Add hazelnuts and onion. Cook for about 5 minutes until onions are softened and hazelnuts are slightly toasted.

Add cognac and mushrooms. Cook for about 6 minutes until mushrooms are softened. Remove from heat. Add next 8 ingredients. Stir.

Combine pork, veal and parsley in a medium bowl. Add mushroom mixture. Mix well. Cover mixture and chill for at least 30 minutes.

*(continued on next page)*

## Tip

If suet is not available, you can use the white fatty parts from a thick side of bacon. Cut the pieces to cover the top of the tenderloin.

**Pastry Dough:** Combine first 9 ingredients in a medium bowl. Cut in lard until mixture resembles coarse crumbs.

Add egg, water and vinegar, stirring until mixture starts to come together. Form into a ball. Wrap with wax paper. Chill for at least 30 minutes (in hot weather, chill for at least 1 hour).

Preheat oven to 425°F (220°C). Roll out pastry dough on surface lightly dusted with sweet rice flour. Roll the dough to a size that will enclose beef tenderloin. Place tenderloin on dough. Cover all sides of tenderloin with ground meat. Moisten edges of dough with water. Gently wrap dough over tenderloin, and pinch all edges to seal. Brush dough with egg white. Transfer to ungreased baking sheet. Bake in oven for about 40 minutes until pastry is golden and ground meat is fully cooked. Let stand for 5 to 8 minutes. Cut into 1/2 to 1 inch (12 mm to 2.5 cm) slices with a sharp serrated meat knife.

*1 serving: 1149 Calories; 69 g Total Fat (17 g Mono, 2 g Poly, 27 g Sat); 303 mg Cholesterol; 38 g Carbohydrate; 3 g Fibre; 87 g Protein; 1007 mg Sodium*

1/2 lb (225 g) lean
**ground pork**

1/2 lb (225 g) lean
**ground veal**

1/4 cup (60 mL) chopped
**fresh parsley**

## Pastry Dough

1 cup (250 mL) white
**rice flour**

1/2 cup (125 mL) sweet
**rice flour**

1/2 cup (125 mL) tapioca
**starch**

1/4 cup (60 mL) pea starch

1 Tbsp (15 mL) pea fibre 80

1 Tbsp (15 mL) sugar

1 1/2 tsp (7 mL) xanthan
**gum**

1 tsp (5 mL) baking powder

1 tsp (5 mL) salt

3/4 cup (175 mL) lard

1 large egg, fork-beaten

2 Tbsp (30 mL) water

2 Tbsp (30 mL) vinegar

1 egg white (large),
lightly beaten

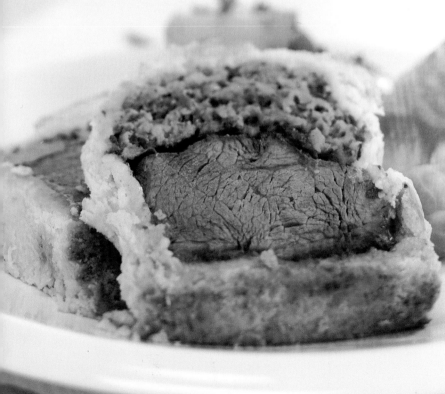

# Meatloaf

## Serves 6 to 8

Pretty much a universal dish, and there are so many variations. In Germany, meatloaf is also known as *Falscher Hase* or "Mock Hare," which refers to its shape if formed freely on a baking pan. Serve with potatoes and vegetables. You can serve meatloaf leftovers on bread as you would a cold cut.

**1 1/2 day-old gluten-free white buns**

**3 to 4 Tbsp (45 to 60 mL) grated onion**

**2 large eggs**

**4 to 6 green onions, chopped**

**1 tsp (5 mL) dried marjoram**

**1 tsp (5 mL) dried thyme**

**1/4 tsp (1 mL) salt**

**1/4 to 1/2 tsp (1 to 2 mL) pepper**

**3/4 lb (340 g) lean ground beef**

**3/4 lb (340 g) lean ground pork**

**1/2 to 1 cup (125 to 250 mL) tomato sauce (optional)**

Preheat oven to 350°F (175°C). Grease a 9 x 5 inch (23 x 12.5 cm) loaf pan. Soak buns in enough water to submerge the buns, just until soft, about 1–3 minutes. Remove buns from water and squeeze gently to remove excess water.

Break buns into pieces and combine with next 7 ingredients in a medium bowl. Add beef and pork. Mix well. Press mixture evenly into prepared loaf pan.

Cover meat with tomato sauce, if desired. Bake, uncovered, in oven for 45 to 50 minutes until fully cooked and internal temperature reaches 160°F (71°C).

*1 serving*: 238 Calories; 14 g Total Fat (4 g Mono, 1 g Poly, 4 g Sat); 113 mg Cholesterol; 8 g Carbohydrate; 1 g Fibre; 16 g Protein; 214 mg Sodium

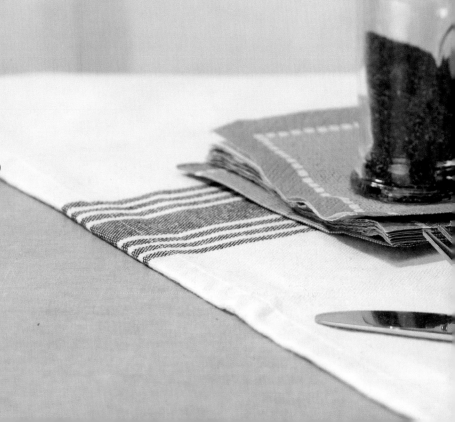

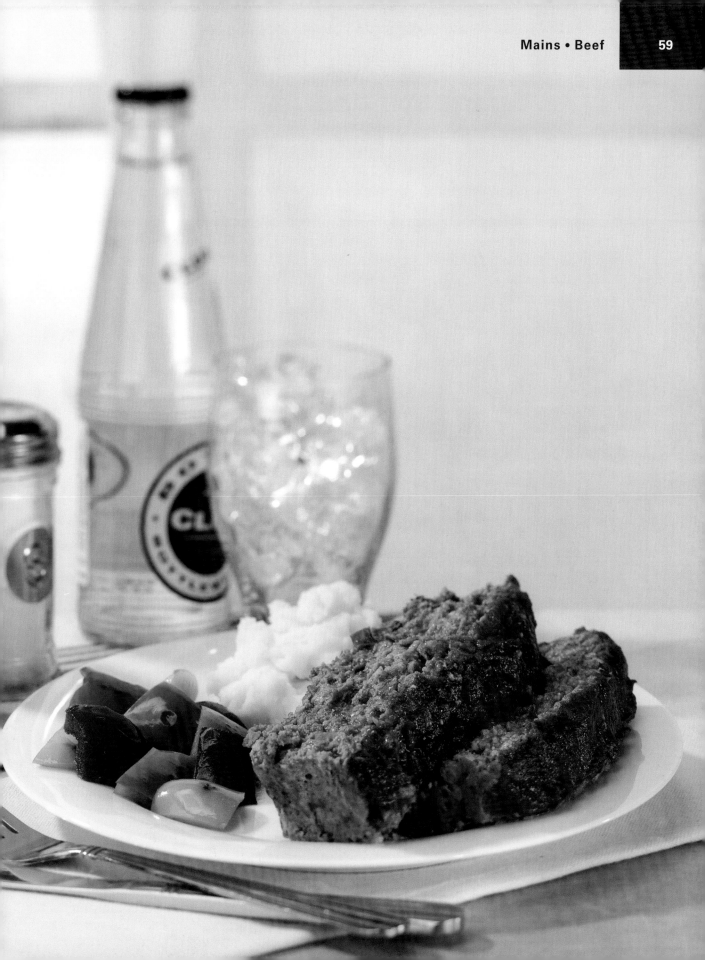

# Spaghetti and Meatballs

## Serves 6 to 8

On top of spaghetti, all covered with cheese, sat a big meatball, fat and all pleased.

**3/4 cup (175 mL) gluten-free dry bread crumbs**

**3 to 4 Tbsp (45 to 60 mL) finely grated onion**

**2 large eggs**

**1 tsp (5 mL) dried rosemary, crushed**

**1/4 tsp (1 mL) salt**

**1/4 to 1/2 tsp (1 to 2 mL) pepper**

**1 1/2 lbs (680 g) lean ground beef**

**12 oz (340 g) gluten-free corn spaghetti**

**2 to 3 cups (500 to 750 mL) gluten-free pasta sauce**

**1/4 to 1/2 cup (60 to 125 mL) grated mozzarella (or Cheddar) cheese**

**Parmesan cheese, to taste**

Preheat oven to 350°F (175°C). Combine first 6 ingredients in a medium bowl. Add beef. Mix well. Roll mixture into balls, using about 1/4 cup (60 mL) for each ball. Arrange meatballs in single layer on ungreased baking sheet with sides. Bake in oven for 20 to 25 minutes until fully cooked and internal temperature reaches 160°F (71°C).

Prepare spaghetti according to package directions. Warm up pasta sauce. Serve meatballs and pasta sauce over spaghetti. Top with cheese and Parmesan cheese.

*1 serving:* 564 Calories; 21 g Total Fat (8 g Mono, 1 g Poly, 7 g Sat); 142 mg Cholesterol; 55 g Carbohydrate; 7 g Fibre; 31 g Protein; 555 mg Sodium

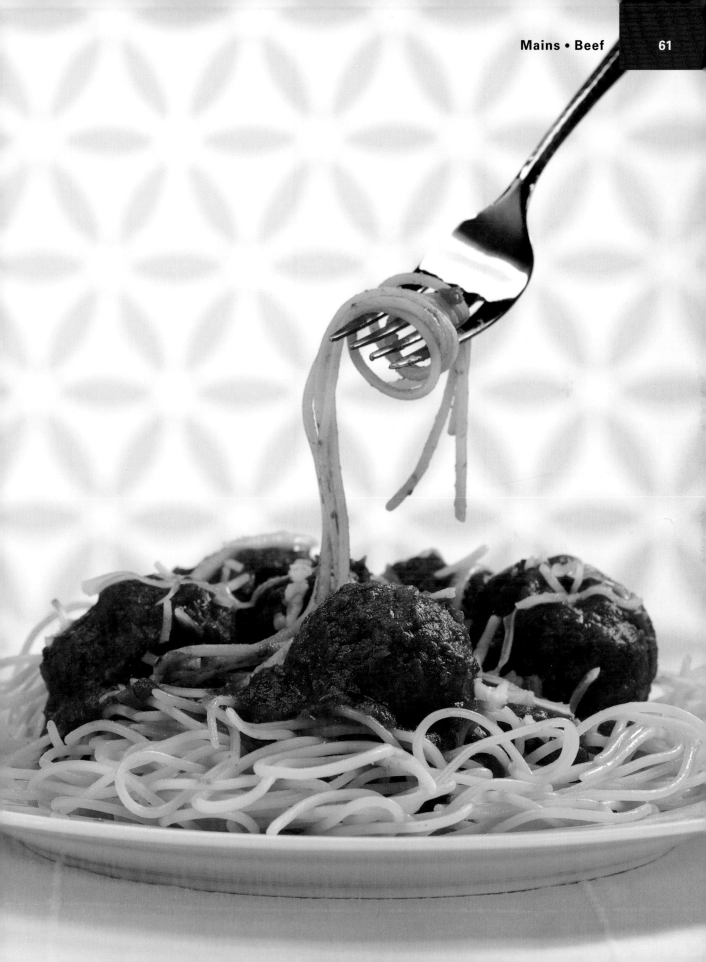

# Koenigsberger Klopse

## Serves 6 to 8

A very distinct meatball variety with capers and white wine in a white sauce. It's especially delicious served with Spaetzle (see page 142) or potatoes, along with red cabbage or your favourite vegetables.

| | |
|---|---|
| **1 1/2 day-old gluten-free white buns** | Soak buns in enough water to submerge the buns, just until soft, about 1–3 minutes. Press to remove excess water. |
| **3 to 4 Tbsp (45 to 60 mL) grated onion** | Combine buns pieces and next 4 ingredients in a medium bowl. Add beef and pork. Cover mixture and chill in refrigerator for about 1 hour. Roll into balls, using about 1/4 cup (60 mL) for each meatball. |
| **2 large eggs, fork-beaten** | |
| **1/4 tsp (1 mL) salt** | |
| **1/4 to 1/2 tsp (1 to 2 mL) pepper** | |

**1 1/2 day-old gluten-free white buns**

Soak buns in enough water to submerge the buns, just until soft, about 1–3 minutes. Press to remove excess water.

**3 to 4 Tbsp (45 to 60 mL) grated onion**

**2 large eggs, fork-beaten**

**1/4 tsp (1 mL) salt**

**1/4 to 1/2 tsp (1 to 2 mL) pepper**

Combine buns pieces and next 4 ingredients in a medium bowl. Add beef and pork. Cover mixture and chill in refrigerator for about 1 hour. Roll into balls, using about 1/4 cup (60 mL) for each meatball.

**3/4 lb (340 g) lean ground beef**

**3/4 lb (340 g) lean ground pork**

**1 1/2 cups (375 mL) chicken broth**

Pour chicken broth into a medium pot. Bring to a boil. Reduce heat to medium-low. Add meatballs, evenly spaced apart. Cook for 15 minutes until meatballs are fully cooked and internal temperature reaches 160°F (71°C). Transfer meatballs with slotted spoon to a bowl. Cover to keep warm. Set chicken broth aside.

**1/3 cup (75 mL) butter**

**1/4 to 1/3 cup (60 to 75 mL) gluten-free all-purpose flour (see page 9)**

**1/2 cup (125 mL) white wine**

**2 1/2 cups (625 mL) milk**

**3 Tbsp (45 mL) capers**

Melt butter in a separate pot. Add flour. Heat and stir for 1 minute. Slowly add white wine and milk, stirring constantly until smooth. Add capers. Stir. Simmer for 3 to 5 minutes until slightly thickened. Depending on desired consistency of sauce, add 1/4 cup (60 mL) or more of hot chicken broth. Add meatballs to sauce.

*1 serving: 416 Calories; 25 g Total Fat (7 g Mono, 1 g Poly, 12 g Sat); 144 mg Cholesterol; 19 g Carbohydrate; 1 g Fibre; 21 g Protein; 622 mg Sodium*

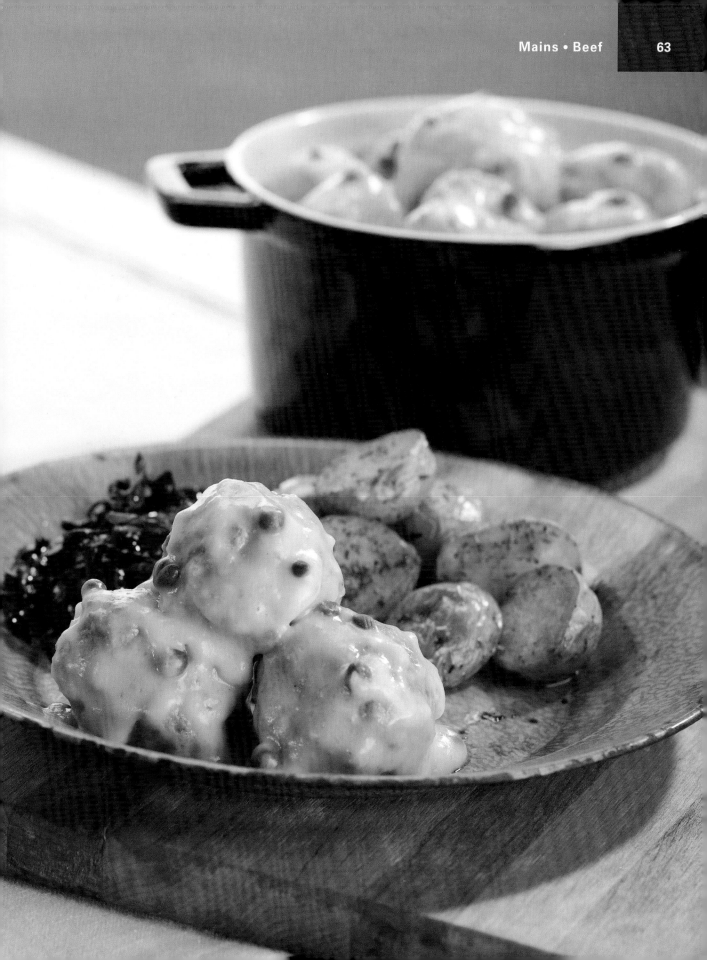

# Beef Teriyaki

## Serves 6

A simple and quick meat and vegetable dish. Easy to prepare and good for lunch or dinner. Serve with green beans and mixed brown rice. Mixed brown rice is available at most grocery stores. It provides a neutral yet flavourful taste and looks good on the plate.

1/3 cup (75 mL) gluten-free teriyaki sauce (see page 156)

1 Tbsp (15 mL) gluten-free all-purpose flour (see page 9)

1 Tbsp (15 mL) olive oil

2 lbs (900 g) beef tenderloin roast, sliced and cut into thin strips

2 to 3 Tbsp (30 to 45 mL) butter

1/2 to 3/4 cup (125 to 175 mL) gluten-free teriyaki sauce

Combine first 3 ingredients in a medium bowl. Add beef strips. Chill, covered, in refrigerator for 40 minutes or overnight. Discard remaining marinade.

Heat butter in a large frying pan on medium-high. Add beef strips. Cook for 3 to 4 minutes until desired doneness. Serve with teriyaki sauce on the side.

*1 serving:* 467 Calories; 34 g Total Fat (15 g Mono, 1 g Poly, 14 g Sat); 113 mg Cholesterol; 4 g Carbohydrate; 0 g Fibre; 31 g Protein; 625 mg Sodium

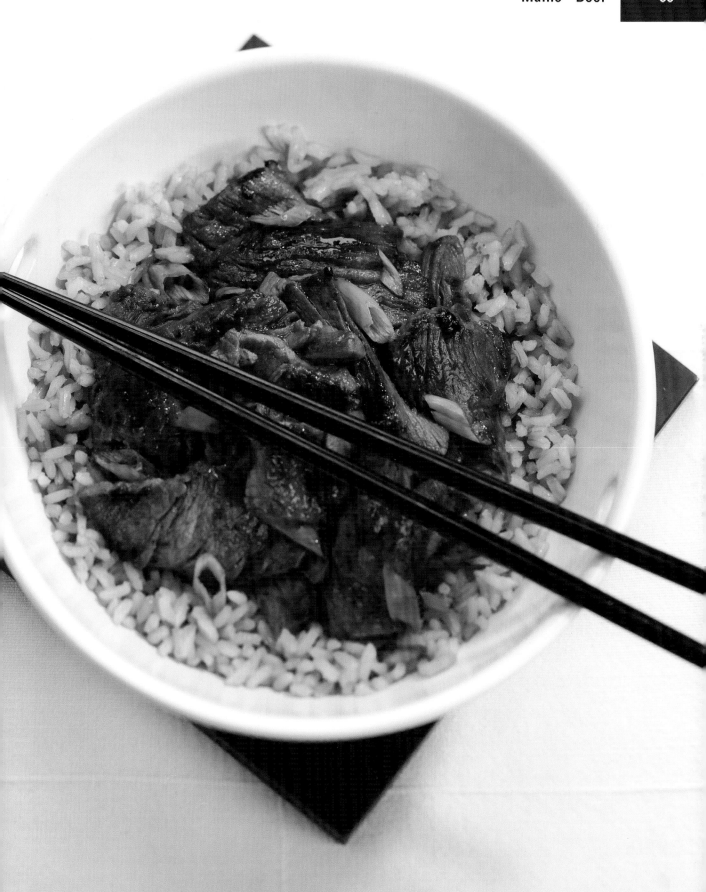

# Beef Pot Pie

## Serves 4 to 6

A tender meat and vegetable filling cooked in red wine and baked between a flaky pastry shell. Use a pre-made gluten-free pastry dough, or follow the pastry recipe below.

## Pastry Crust

1 cup (250 mL) white rice flour

1/2 cup (125 mL) sweet rice flour

1/2 cup (125 mL) tapioca starch

1/4 cup (60 mL) pea starch

1 Tbsp (15 mL) pea fibre 80

1 Tbsp (15 mL) sugar

1 1/2 tsp (7 mL) xanthan gum

1 tsp (5 mL) baking powder

1 tsp (5 mL) salt

3/4 cup (175 mL) lard

1 large egg

2 Tbsp (30 mL) vinegar

2 Tbsp (30 mL) water, approximately (if necessary)

(continued on next page)

**Pastry Crust:** Preheat oven to 350°F (175°C). Combine first 9 ingredients in a large bowl. Cut in lard until mixture resembles coarse crumbs.

Add egg, vinegar and water, if necessary (only add water if dough is too dry to make a pliable pie dough). Stir until pastry mixture starts to come together. Do not over mix. Dust hands with sweet rice flour. Divide dough into 2 portions. Roll out one portion to about 1/8 inch (3 mm) thickness and line a 9-inch (23 cm) pie plate, or press one portion directly into pie plate.

**Filling:** Heat cooking oil in a large pot on medium. Add beef. Cook for 10 minutes, stirring occasionally, until browned on all sides. Reduce heat to low. Add wine. Cook, covered, for 12 to 15 minutes until liquid is evaporated.

Add remaining 3 ingredients. Cook for 10 to 12 more minutes, stirring occasionally, until carrots are softened. Spread mixture into pie crust. Roll out second portion of dough to about 1/8 inch (3 mm) thickness. Cover pie with remaining pastry. Trim and crimp decorative edge to seal. Cut several small slits in top pie crust. Bake on middle rack of preheated oven for 35 to 45 minutes until pastry is golden and filling is bubbling. Remove from oven and place pie on wire rack to cool for 10 to 12 minutes before serving.

*1 serving: 969 Calories; 60 g Total Fat (7 g Mono, 2 g Poly, 23 g Sat); 115 mg Cholesterol; 78 g Carbohydrate; 5 g Fibre; 19 g Protein; 859 mg Sodium*

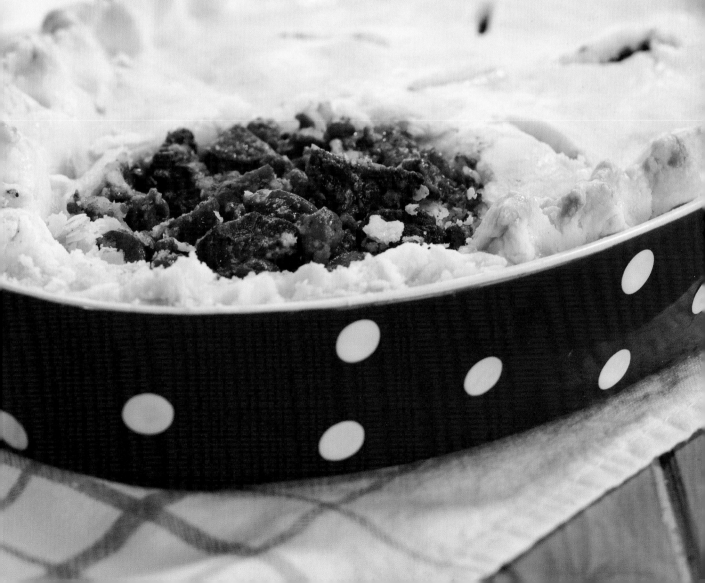

## Filling

1 to 2 Tbsp (15 to 30 mL) cooking oil

1/2 lb (225 g) beef roast, cut into 1/4 to 1/2 inch (6 to 12 mm) cubes

1 cup (250 mL) red wine

3/4 cup (175 mL) gravy (see page 154)

1/2 cup (125 mL) fresh (or frozen) peas

1/2 cup (125 mL) thinly sliced carrots

# Chili Con Carne in a Bread Bowl

## Serves 6

A classic bean and meat dish served in hollowed-out gluten-free bread instead of a bowl. I use the following bread recipe, but you could use any unsliced gluten-free bread or bun you like. Make the bread a few hours or a day ahead of time so it can firm up a bit. Serve chili with yogurt or sour cream.

## Bread Bowl

1/4 cup (60 mL) warm water

1 Tbsp (15 mL) active dry yeast

2 tsp (10 mL) sugar

1 1/2 cups (375 mL) tapioca starch

1 1/2 cups (375 mL) white rice flour

1/4 cup (60 mL) whey powder

2 Tbsp (30 mL) pea fibre 80

2 Tbsp (30 mL) sugar

4 tsp (20 mL) xanthan gum

1 tsp (5 mL) dough improver (see page 9)

1 tsp (5 mL) salt

1 1/4 cups (300 mL) water

4 egg whites, room temperature

## Chili Con Carne

3 Tbsp (45 mL) butter

1 large onion, finely chopped

4 garlic cloves, minced

(continued on next page)

**Bread Bowl:** Preheat oven to 375°F (190°C). Place first 3 ingredients in a small bowl. Let stand for 10 minutes until foamy.

Mix next 8 ingredients in a large bowl.

Mix water and egg whites in a separate bowl. Add egg white mixture and yeast mixture to flour mixture. Stir until a smooth batter is formed. Turn out onto a surface lightly dusted with white rice flour. Divide dough into 6 equal portions. Roll portions into balls. Arrange balls, not touching, on a greased baking sheet. Smooth the dough ball surface with a wet spatula. Place in a warm place and cover with a damp towel. Let dough rise for 20 to 30 minutes until about doubled in size. Bake on middle rack of preheated oven for 25 to 30 minutes until buns sound hollow when tapped. Remove from oven and place on a wire rack to cool. Once cooled, scoop out the centre of each bun, leaving enough crust to create a bowl for the chili con carne.

**Chili Con Carne:** Heat butter in a large frying pan on medium-high. Add onion and garlic. Cook for 5 to 10 minutes, stirring occasionally, until softened. Add next 3 ingredients. Scramble-fry for 9 to 12 minutes until meat is no longer pink. Drain. Transfer beef mixture to a medium pot.

(continued on next page)

Add next 9 ingredients. Cook, covered, on medium for about 1 hour, stirring occasionally, until thickened.

If a thicker chili is desired, combine 1 to 2 Tbsp (15 to 30 mL) gluten-free all-purpose flour (see page 9) and 1/3 cup (75 mL) water in a small bowl. Slowly add to beef mixture, stirring constantly. Cook for 5 minutes. Scoop chili into bread bowls to 3/4 full. Break bread crust to eat chili or use a spoon.

*1 serving:* 918 Calories; 28 g Total Fat (11 g Mono, 1 g Poly, 12 g Sat); 111 mg Cholesterol; 106 g Carbohydrate; 20 g Fibre; 47 g Protein; 1609 mg Sodium

**2 lbs (900 g) lean ground beef**

**1 tsp (5 mL) salt**

**1/4 tsp (1 mL) pepper**

**1 x 28 oz (796 mL) can of diced tomatoes**

**2 x 14 oz (398 mL) cans of red kidney beans, rinsed and drained**

**3/4 cup (175 mL) thinly sliced carrots**

**1/2 cup (125 mL) corn**

**1/2 cup (125 mL) thinly sliced celery**

**1 to 2 Tbsp (15 to 30 mL) chili powder**

**1 1/2 tsp (7 mL) gluten-free tamari sauce**

**1 tsp (5 mL) dried oregano**

**1 tsp (5 mL) paprika**

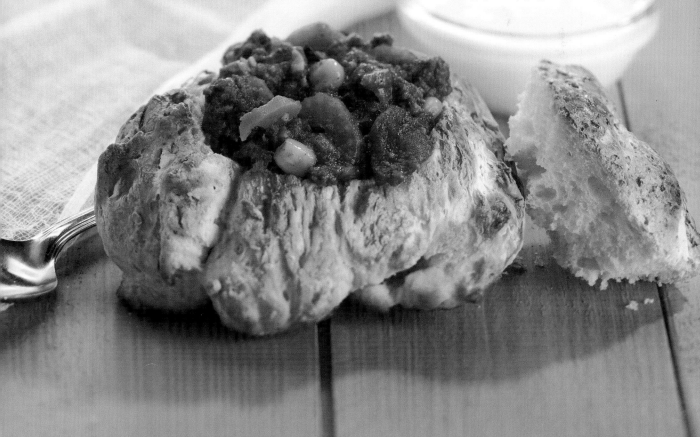

# Lasagna

## Serves 8 to 12

This layered pasta dish is a favourite in our house and is simple to make. You can use premade gluten-free lasagna noodles, or try your hand at the pasta recipe below and make it from scratch. I like to bake this lasagna the day before and chill in the refrigerator so it sets firm. I reheat the lasagna the next day, covered with foil, in the oven at 325°F (160°C) for 20 to 25 minutes, or microwave individual servings for 3 to 4 minutes.

## Pasta

1 cup (250 mL) yellow corn flour

1/4 cup (60 mL) pea starch

1/4 cup (60 mL) rice flour

1 to 2 Tbsp (15 to 30 mL) pea fibre 80

2 tsp (10 mL) xanthan gum

1 tsp (5 mL) fine sea salt

1 tsp (5 mL) guar gum

4 egg yolks (large)

2 large eggs, room temperature

## Lasagna

2 lbs (900 g) lean ground beef

2 to 3 cups (500 to 750 mL) gluten-free pasta sauce

1/4 to 1/3 cup (60 to 75 mL) grated Parmesan cheese

1 lb (454 g) grated mozzarella cheese

2 cups (500 mL) dry curd cottage cheese

**Pasta:** Mix first 7 ingredients together in a heavy-duty mixer.

Add egg yolks and eggs. Mix on medium with a paddle attachment for 2 to 3 minutes until well blended. Dough will feel pliable but not too soft.

If you're using a pasta machine, follow the manufacturer's instructions, understanding that gluten-free dough will be slightly stickier and less pliable. I roll the dough out to about 1/2 inch (12 mm) thickness between pieces of parchment paper before running through the pasta machine. Use a bit of pea starch for dusting if necessary to prevent sticking.

To make lasagna noodles without a pasta machine, divide dough into small pieces about 1 1/2 to 2 inches (4 to 5 cm), or the size of a ping-pong ball. Lightly dust surface with pea starch. Roll out each piece as thin as possible. Cut into 9 x 13 inch (23 x 33 cm) sheets or cut into 9 x 2 inch (23 x 5 cm) strips. Makes 9 to 12 lasagna sheets.

**Lasagna:** Preheat oven to 350°F (175°C). Scramble-fry beef in a large frying pan until no longer pink. Add pasta sauce and stir. To assemble, layer ingredients in ungreased 9 x 13 inch (23 x 33 cm) baking dish as follows:

• 1/4 meat sauce

• 1/3 Parmesan cheese

• layer of pasta

• 1/4 meat sauce

• 1/3 Parmesan cheese

• 1/3 mozzarella cheese

*(continued on next page)*

- layer of pasta

- 1/4 meat sauce

- cottage cheese

- 1/3 mozzarella cheese

- layer of pasta

- 1/4 meat sauce

- 1/3 mozzarella cheese

- 1/3 Parmesan cheese

Cover pan with greased foil. Bake in preheated oven for about 45 minutes. Remove from oven and let stand for 10 to 15 minutes before serving.

*1 serving: 633 Calories; 33 g Total Fat (12 g Mono, 1 g Poly, 15 g Sat); 257 mg Cholesterol; 27 g Carbohydrate; 4 g Fibre; 47 g Protein; 1012 mg Sodium*

*I use my homemade uncooked noodles in lasagna, making sure to cover them with sauce. If you'd like to cook your pasta first, remember that fresh pasta cooks faster than dry pasta—typically about 5 minutes to reach* al dente *in boiling salted water.*

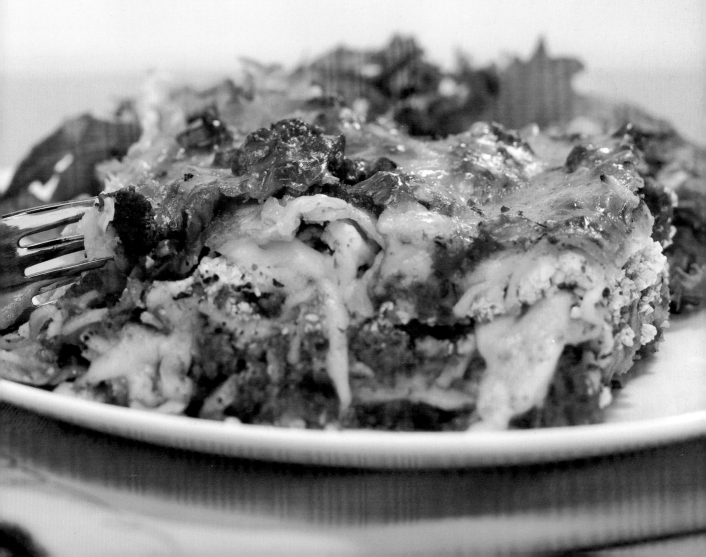

# Chicken Stew with Rice

## Serves 6 to 8

A thick, creamy chicken stew, similar to a fricassee-style dish, served over whole-grain rice. Double the recipe if you'd like to freeze some for later use.

2 1/2 cups (625 mL) water

pinch of salt

1 cup (250 mL) whole-grain rice

Combine water and salt in a pot and bring to a boil. Add rice. Reduce heat to low. Cook, covered, according to package directions or for 35 to 40 minutes, without stirring, until rice is tender. Set aside.

2 Tbsp (30 mL) cooking oil

3 lbs (1.4 kg) boneless, skinless chicken breasts, cut into 3/4 inch (2 cm) cubes

1 tsp (5 mL) gluten-free soy sauce

1 tsp (5 mL) gluten-free teriyaki sauce (see page 156)

1/4 tsp (1 mL) salt

1/8 tsp (0.5 mL) pepper

Heat cooking oil and next 5 ingredients in a large frying pan on medium. Heat and stir for 5 to 8 minutes until chicken is no longer pink.

Add next 4 ingredients. Heat and stir for 1 to 2 minutes.

Heat first amount of chicken broth on medium until hot but not boiling. Carefully add chicken and vegetable mixture to broth. Simmer, uncovered, on low for 25 minutes. Add broccoli. Simmer for 5 minutes. Remove from heat.

4 medium carrots, cut into 1/4 inch (6 mm) slices

3 to 4 celery stalks, cut into 1/4 inch (6 mm) slices

2 to 3 medium potatoes, peeled and cubed

1 medium onion, cut into 1/4 inch (6 mm) slices

In a small bowl, add flour to second amount of chicken broth, constantly stirring. Add whipping cream. Add mixture to chicken stew, constantly stirring. Bring to a boil. Heat and stir for 1 minute. Serve stew over rice.

*1 serving:* 442 Calories; 12 g Total Fat (5 g Mono, 2 g Poly, 4 g Sat); 174 mg Cholesterol; 27 g Carbohydrate; 3 g Fibre; 57 g Protein; 679 mg Sodium

*(continued on next page)*

2 3/4 to 3 1/4 cup (675 to 800 mL) chicken broth

1 cup (250 mL) frozen chopped broccoli

1/4 to 1/3 cup (60 to 75 mL) gluten-free all-purpose flour (see page 9)

3/4 cup (175 mL) chicken broth

1/3 cup (75 mL) whipping cream

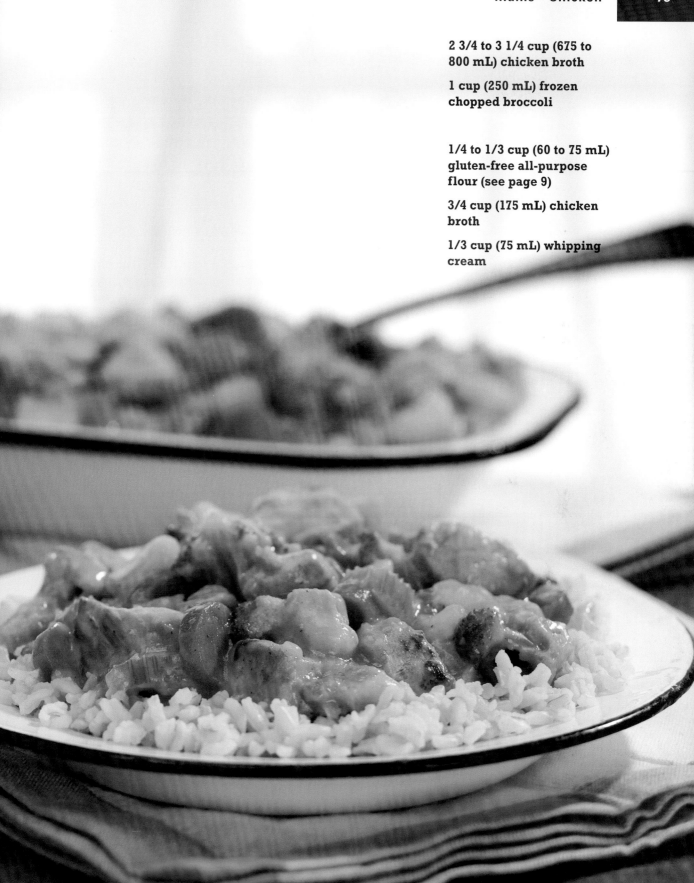

# Coq au Vin

## Serves 6 to 8

The name itself is enough reason to try this classic French dish—it kind of rolls off your tongue. This dish takes a bit of effort, but it's a great way to serve chicken. While cooking, help yourself to a glass or two of the red *vin* that you will add to the *coq*. If you can't find fresh herbs, you can replace them with 1/2 tsp (2 mL) dried herbs each. Serve over Spaetzle (see page 142) or pasta.

**5 to 8 low-sodium bacon slices, chopped**

**3 1/2 lbs (1.6 kg) bone-in chicken thighs and drumsticks**

**3 to 4 Tbsp (45 to 60 mL) gluten-free all-purpose flour (see page 9)**

**1 1/2 to 2 cups (375 to 500 mL) chicken broth**

**1 1/2 to 2 cups (375 to 500 mL) red wine (pinot noir or burgundy)**

**4 to 6 garlic cloves, minced**

**2 bay leaves**

**1 Tbsp (15 mL) tomato paste**

**1/2 tsp (2 mL) salt**

**1/4 tsp (1 mL) pepper**

**1 to 2 sprigs of fresh thyme**

**1 to 2 sprigs of fresh marjoram**

**1 to 2 sprigs of fresh parsley**

**1/2 lb (225 g) mushrooms, sliced**

**2 cups (500 mL) carrots, sliced**

**1 large onion, diced**

Preheat oven to 350°F (175°C). Cook bacon in a large Dutch oven on medium until crisp. Transfer bacon with a slotted spoon to a paper towel–lined plate to drain. Add chicken pieces to hot bacon drippings, in batches if necessary, and cook for 5 to 8 minutes on each side until browned. Transfer chicken with slotted spoon to plate.

Add flour to bacon drippings. Cook, stirring, until bubbles form. Add next 10 ingredients. Cook for 3 to 7 minutes, stirring constantly, until mixture thickens. Remove from heat.

Add chicken and next 3 ingredients. Stir. Bake, covered, in preheated oven for 80 minutes. Remove bay leaves before serving.

*1 serving:* 551 Calories; 26 g Total Fat (11 g Mono, 5 g Poly, 8 g Sat); 211 mg Cholesterol; 16 g Carbohydrate; 2 g Fibre; 55 g Protein; 621 mg Sodium

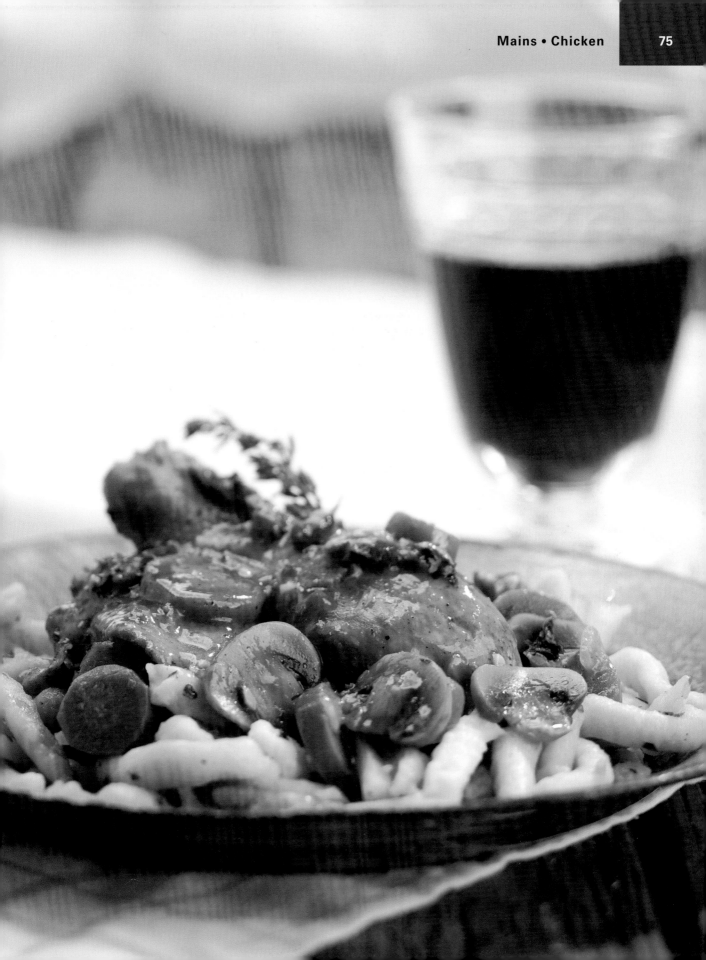

# Chicken Cordon Bleu

## Serves 6

A timeless classic well worth the extra time. The combination of tender chicken with melted cheese and crunchy crust is complimented by a creamy white wine sauce. Serve with rice or vegetables.

### Cordon Bleu

6 x 4 to 6 oz (113 to 170 g) boneless, skinless chicken breast halves

1 tsp (5 mL) salt

1 tsp (5 mL) pepper

3 provolone cheese slices, halved

6 Swiss cheese slices

6 thin deli smoked ham slices

1/2 cup (125 mL) gluten-free all-purpose flour (see page 9)

1 1/2 cups (375 mL) gluten-free herb bread crumbs (see page 148) or panko crumbs

2 tsp (10 mL) Italian seasoning (optional)

2 large eggs, fork-beaten

6 to 8 Tbsp (90 to 120 mL) butter

*(continued on next page)*

**Cordon Bleu:** Preheat oven to 350°F (175°C). Spray a baking sheet with cooking spray. Place each chicken breast between 2 sheets of plastic wrap on cutting board. Pound with mallet or rolling pin to about 1/4 inch (6 mm) thickness. Sprinkle with salt and pepper.

Top each chicken breast with provolone cheese, Swiss cheese and ham. Roll up each chicken breast tightly. Fasten each roll with a wooden pick.

Place flour in a small shallow dish. Combine bread crumbs and seasoning in a separate small shallow dish. Place eggs in separate dish. Press each chicken roll into flour until coated. Dip in egg, then press into bread crumb mixture. Discard any remaining flour, egg and bread crumb mixture. Place chicken rolls, seam-side down, on baking sheet. Put 1 1/4 Tbsp (20 mL) butter on top of each chicken breast. Bake in preheated oven for 35 to 40 minutes until internal temperature of chicken reaches 170°F (77°C). Temperature of stuffing should reach at least 165°F (74°C).

*(continued on next page)*

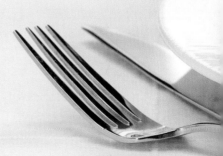

**Sauce:** Combine first amount of cream and cornstarch. Set aside.

Combine remaining 8 ingredients in a medium saucepan on medium-low. Bring to a gentle boil, stirring occasionally. Add cornstarch mixture. Return to a boil. Cook, stirring constantly, until thickened. Pour sauce over chicken and serve.

*1 serving*: 720 Calories; 43 g Total Fat (11 g Mono, 2 g Poly, 26 g Sat); 256 mg Cholesterol; 29 g Carbohydrate; 1 g Fibre; 48 g Protein; 1466 mg Sodium

**Sauce**

1/2 cup (125 mL) half-and-half cream

2 to 3 Tbsp (30 to 45 mL) cornstarch

1 cup (250 mL) chicken broth

1 cup (250 mL) whipping cream

1/2 cup (125 mL) half-and-half cream

1/2 cup (125 mL) white wine

1 tsp (5 mL) ground marjoram

1/2 tsp (2 mL) salt

1/2 tsp (2 mL) pepper

1/4 tsp (1 mL) crushed garlic

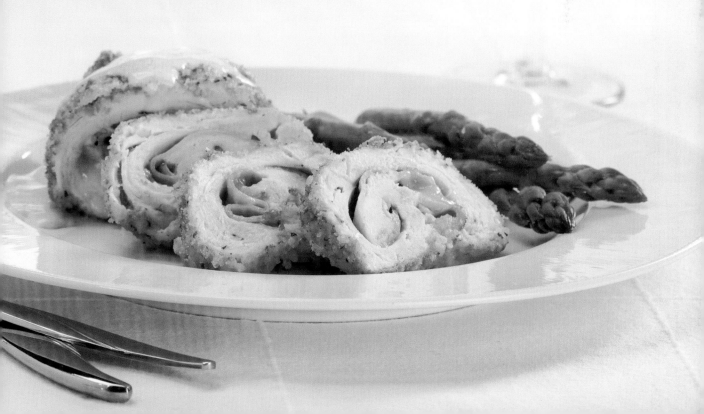

# Chicken Fingers

## Makes 2 dozen

Crispy coated chicken strips with balanced seasonings. Served with a plum sauce or creamy dressing, these make good appetizers or snacks.

**6 x 4 to 6 oz (113 to 170 g) boneless, skinless chicken breast halves**

**2 cups (500 mL) crushed gluten-free cornflakes cereal**

**1 Tbsp (15 mL) paprika**

**2 tsp (10 mL) poultry seasoning**

**1 tsp (5 mL) pepper**

**1 tsp (5 mL) salt**

**2 egg whites (large), fork-beaten**

Preheat oven to 350°F (175°C). Cut chicken breasts into strips 3/4 inch (2 cm) wide.

Combine next 5 ingredients in a bowl. Transfer mixture to a large resealable freezer bag. Dip chicken strips in egg whites until coated. Drop coated chicken strips into resealable bag. Seal bag and shake until chicken is coated. Place chicken on an ungreased baking sheet. Bake in oven for 20 to 25 minutes until crispy and no longer pink inside. Serve with your favourite dipping sauce.

*1 finger:* 65 Calories; 0 g Total Fat (0 g Mono, 0 g Poly, 0 g Sat); 16 mg Cholesterol; 7 g Carbohydrate; 0 g Fibre; 7 g Protein; 177 mg Sodium

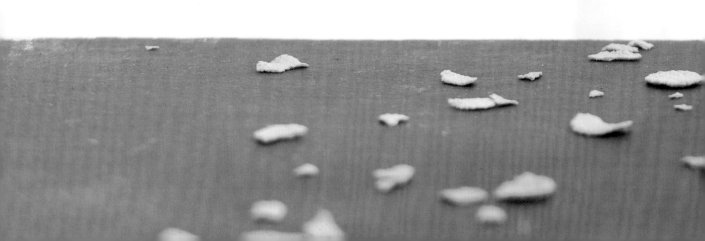

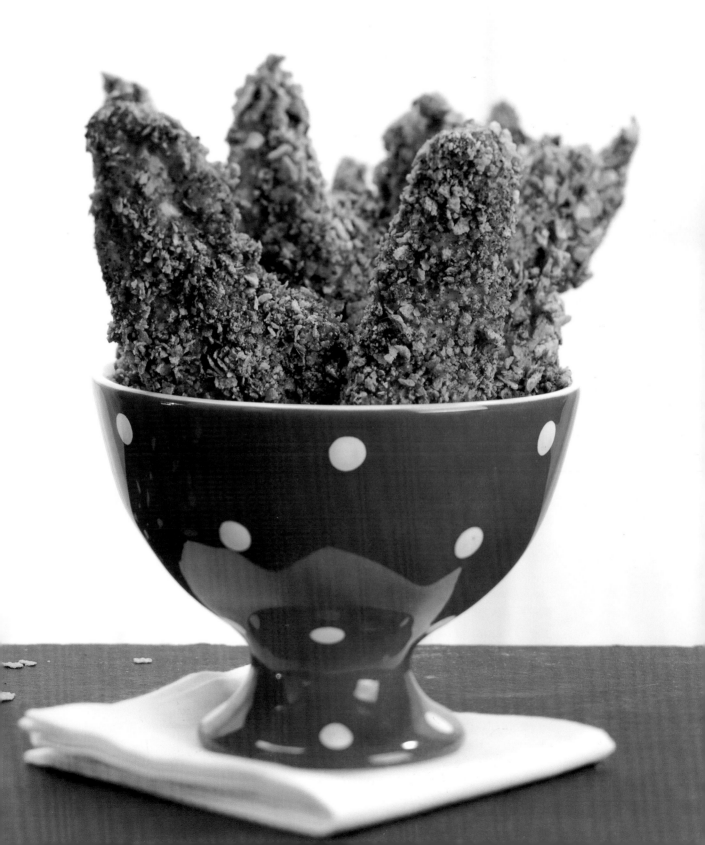

# Chicken Drumsticks with Sweet Potato Fries

### Serves 6

These drumsticks are coated in classic cornflake crumbs and spices and oven-baked instead of deep-fried. Sweet potato fries make a nice addition.

## Chicken Drumsticks

2 cups (500 mL) crushed gluten-free cornflakes cereal

1/4 cup (60 mL) gluten-free all-purpose flour (see page 9)

1 Tbsp (15 mL) Hungarian paprika

1 tsp (5 mL) cayenne pepper

1 tsp (5 mL) poultry seasoning

1 tsp (5 mL) salt

4 1/2 lbs (2 kg) chicken drumsticks

3/4 cup (175 mL) butter, melted

## Sweet Potato Fries

3 to 4 large sweet potatoes, cut into 1/2 to 3/4 inch (1.2 to 2 cm) wide strips

2 to 3 Tbsp (30 to 45 mL) olive oil

sprinkle of salt

sprinkle of Hungarian paprika

**Chicken Drumsticks:** Preheat oven to 400°F (200°C). Combine first 6 ingredients in a large resealable bag.

Brush drumsticks with butter. Drop into resealable bag. Seal bag and shake until chicken is coated. Place on an ungreased baking sheet. Bake chicken in oven for 35 to 40 minutes until crispy and no longer pink inside.

**Sweet Potato Fries:** Spread sweet potato strips on a greased baking sheet, not overlapping. Brush with olive oil and sprinkle with salt and paprika. Bake in preheated oven for 20 to 25 minutes. Flip fries. Bake for another 10 minutes until crisp.

*1 serving (with fries): 1111 Calories; 71 g Total Fat (26 g Mono, 11 g Poly, 27 g Sat); 337 mg Cholesterol; 51 g Carbohydrate; 4 g Fibre; 64 g Protein; 1112 mg Sodium*

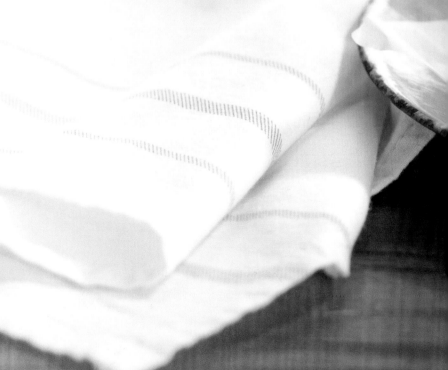

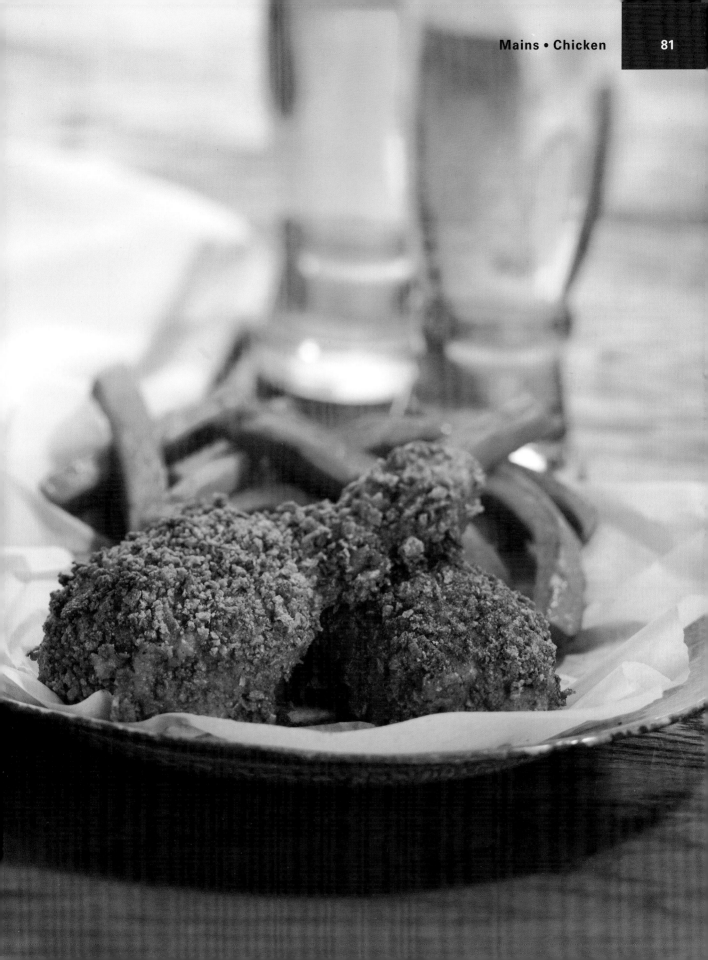

# Curried Chicken

## Serves 6

Curry, fruit, nuts and chicken make for a winning and satisfying combo in this perfectly spiced dish. Serve with broccoli to make a complete meal.

**2 Tbsp (30 mL) cooking oil**

**1 medium red onion, finely chopped**

**1 garlic clove, minced**

**1/2 cup (125 mL) sliced almonds**

**6 x 4 to 6 oz (113 to 170 g) boneless, skinless chicken breast halves, cut into 1/2 inch (12 mm) cubes**

**1 to 2 tsp (5 to 10 mL) curry powder**

**1 tsp (5 mL) paprika**

**1 tsp (5 mL) salt**

**1 tsp (5 mL) pepper**

**1 tsp (5 mL) poultry seasoning**

**1 tsp (5 mL) gluten-free soy sauce**

**1 x 14 oz (398 mL) can of sliced peaches in juice, drained**

**1/2 cup (125 mL) medium shredded coconut**

**1/2 cup (125 mL) plain Greek yogurt**

**1 Tbsp (15 mL) gluten-free all-purpose flour (see page 9)**

Heat cooking oil in a large pot on medium. Add onion and garlic. Cook for 2 to 3 minutes, stirring often, until softened. Add almonds. Cook for 3 to 5 minutes until almonds are slightly browned. Add chicken. Cook for 3 to 5 minutes, stirring constantly, until chicken no longer pink.

Add next 6 ingredients. Stir well.

Add next 4 ingredients. Cook for 10 to 15 minutes, stirring occasionally.

Preheat oven to 400°F (200°C). Combine remaining 4 ingredients in a small bowl. Transfer chicken mixture to a lightly greased 9 x 13 inch (23 x 33 cm) baking dish. Top evenly with cornflakes, sugar and cheese mixture. Bake on middle rack of oven for 15 to 20 minutes until cheese is melted and slightly browned.

*1 serving:* 502 Calories; 17 g Total Fat (6 g Mono, 3 g Poly, 6 g Sat); 78 mg Cholesterol; 53 g Carbohydrate; 4 g Fibre; 34 g Protein; 859 mg Sodium

*(continued on next page)*

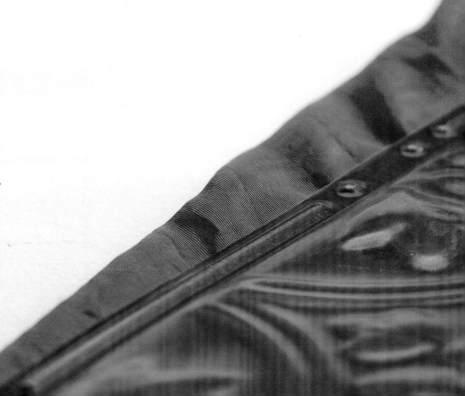

2 cups (500 mL) crushed
gluten-free cornflakes
cereal

1/4 cup (60 mL) brown
sugar, packed

1/4 cup (60 mL) grated
mozzarella cheese

1/4 cup (60 mL) grated
Parmesan cheese

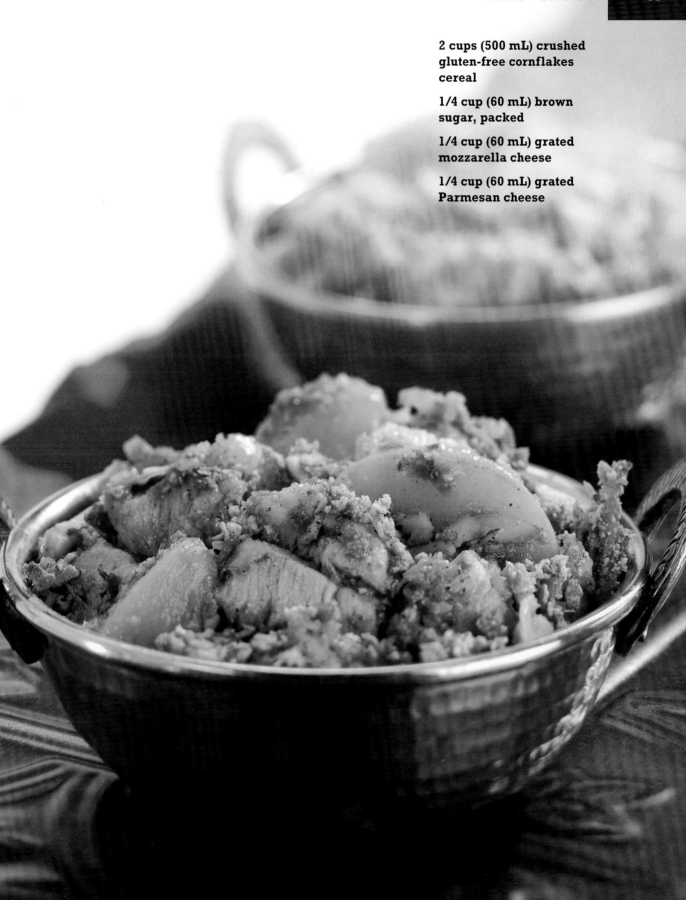

# Chicken Burgers

## Serves 6 to 8

A lighter variation on the traditional hamburger. I use soft hamburger buns from Kinnikinnick Foods.

**3/4 cup (175 mL) gluten-free bread crumbs (see page 9)**

**3 to 4 Tbsp (45 to 60 mL) grated onion**

**2 large eggs, fork-beaten**

**1 tsp (5 mL) poultry seasoning**

**1/4 tsp (1 mL) salt**

**1/4 to 1/2 tsp (1 to 2 mL) pepper**

**1 1/2 lbs (680 g) lean ground chicken**

**6 to 8 gluten-free buns**

**1 Tbsp (15 mL) ranch dressing**

Combine first 6 ingredients in a medium bowl. Add chicken. Mix well. Shape into patties about 3 inches (7.5 cm) wide and 3/4 inch (2 cm) thick. Cook patties in frying pan on medium for 4 to 5 minutes per side until fully cooked and internal temperature reaches 175°F (80°C).

Serve patties on gluten-free buns with ranch dressing and your favourite toppings, like lettuce, tomato, pineapple, avocado or mayo.

*1 serving (with bun): 465 Calories; 27 g Total Fat (1 g Mono, 0 g Poly, 1 g Sat); 156 mg Cholesterol; 30 g Carbohydrate; 3 g Fibre; 24 g Protein; 404 mg Sodium*

*(continued on next page)*

**Frikadellen:** Replace poultry seasoning with thyme. Replace ground chicken with 3/4 lb (340 g) *each* of lean ground beef and lean ground pork. Cook patties until internal temperature reaches 160°F (71°C). Serve on buns, or with potatoes, peas and gravy.

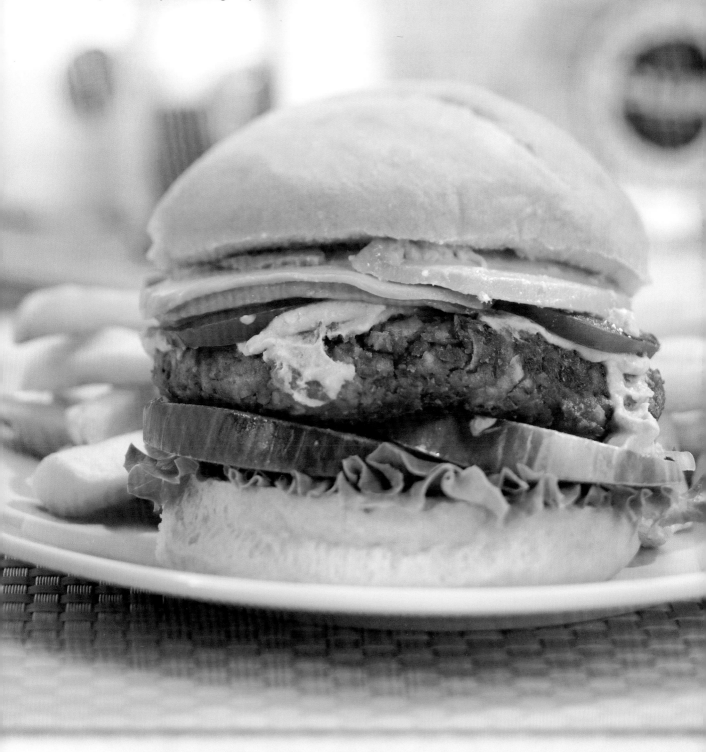

# Breaded Lemon Chicken Breasts

## Serves 6

A simple one-dish main course with a crispy top and soft creamy bottom. The chicken stays tender and juicy. Serve with broccoli.

**2 cups (500 mL) fine gluten-free bread crumbs (see page 9) or panko crumbs**

**1/2 to 1 cup (125 to 250 mL) sweet rice flour**

**grated zest from 2 lemons**

**1 Tbsp (15 mL) paprika**

**2 tsp (10 mL) poultry seasoning**

**1 tsp (5 mL) salt**

**1 tsp (5 mL) pepper**

**1 cup (250 mL) whipping cream**

**6 x 4 to 6 oz (113 to 170 g) boneless, skinless chicken breast halves**

**2 egg whites (large), fork-beaten**

Preheat oven to 350°F (175°C). Combine first 7 ingredients in a medium deep bowl.

Spread whipping cream evenly into a 9 x 13 inch (23 x 33 cm) baking dish. Place chicken on top. Brush chicken with egg whites. Shake crumb mixture over each chicken piece until covered. Bake in oven for 30 to 35 minutes until internal temperature of chicken reaches 170°F (77°C).

*1 serving:* 348 Calories; 14 g Total Fat (4 g Mono, 1 g Poly, 8 g Sat); 125 mg Cholesterol; 24 g Carbohydrate; 1 g Fibre; 32 g Protein; 519 mg Sodium

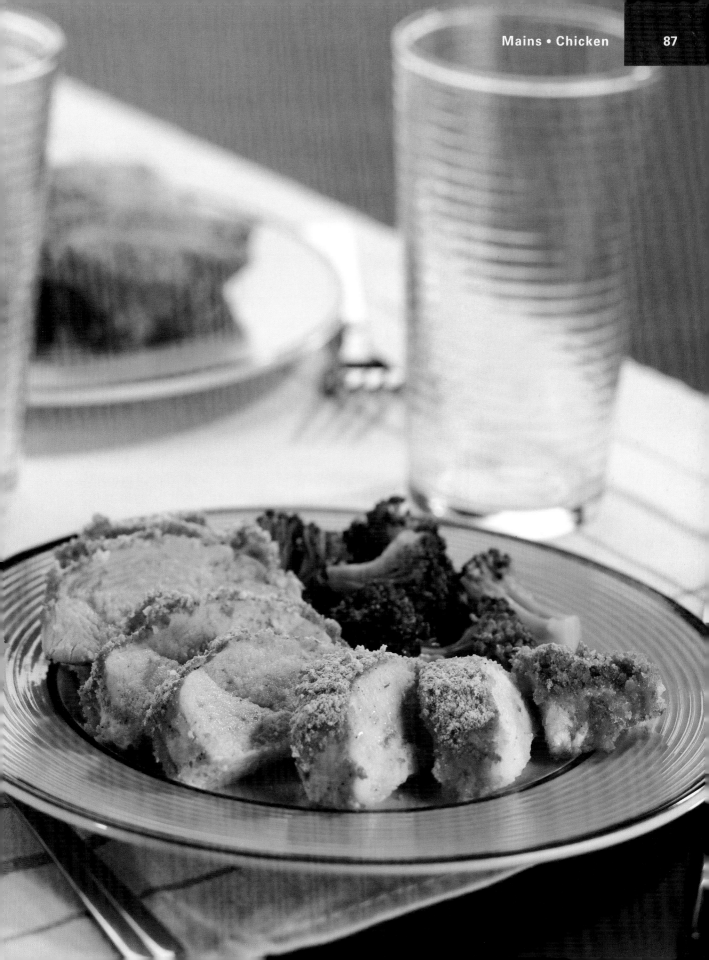

# Fried Chicken

## Serves 6

Crispy, deep-fried chicken, just like your favourite fast-food variety. You can make your own bucket full!

**lard (or shortening or cooking oil), for frying**

**4 1/2 lbs (2 kg) chicken pieces**

**2 cups (500 mL) crushed gluten-free cornflakes cereal**

**1 Tbsp (15 mL) Hungarian paprika**

**1 tsp (5 mL) cayenne pepper**

**1 tsp (5 mL) poultry seasoning**

**1 tsp (5 mL) salt**

**1/2 to 1 cup (125 to 250 mL) gluten-free all-purpose flour (see page 9)**

**2 large eggs, fork-beaten**

Heat lard in deep fryer to 350°F (175°C) as per manufacturer's instructions.

Cut chicken into pieces (you can use drumsticks and bone-in pieces as well).

Combine next 5 ingredients. Transfer to a large resealable freezer bag. Place flour in a small shallow dish. Place eggs in separate shallow dish. Press one chicken piece into flour until coated. Dip chicken piece into egg. Drop chicken into resealable bag. Seal bag and shake until chicken is coated. Transfer chicken piece to a bowl. Repeat process until all chicken pieces have been coated. Discard any remaining flour, egg, and cornflakes mixture. Deep-fry chicken, in batches, for 3 to 5 minutes per batch until crispy and no longer pink inside. Remove each batch to paper towels to drain. Serve with your favourite dipping sauce.

*1 serving:* 719 Calories; 29 g Total Fat (6 g Mono, 5 g Poly, 9 g Sat); 337 mg Cholesterol; 39 g Carbohydrate; 2 g Fibre; 70 g Protein; 944 mg Sodium

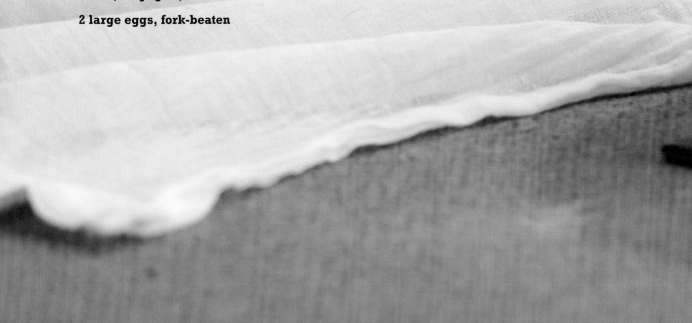

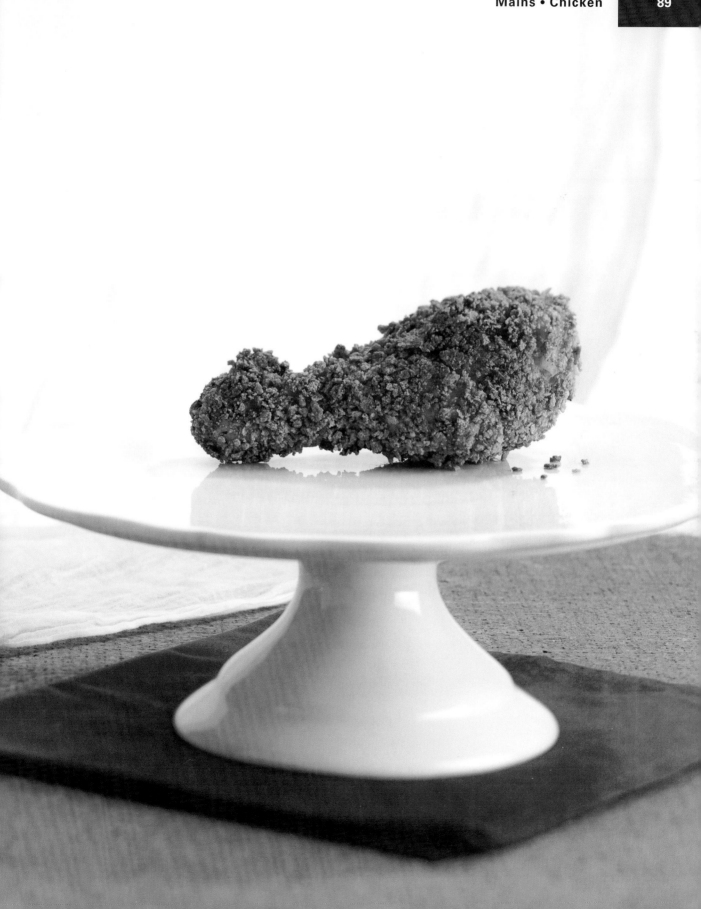

# Chicken Pie

## Serves 4 to 6

A traditional savoury chicken pot pie with a nice blend of meat and vegetables in a creamy sauce. You can use the same recipe to make several individual-sized pies. This pie freezes well.

**2 gluten-free pastry portions, for pie crust (see page 66)**

**1 to 1 1/2 lbs (680 g) boneless, skinless chicken breast, cut into 1/4 to 1/2 inch (6 to 12 mm) cubes**

**1 1/4 cup (300 mL) frozen peas**

**1 1/4 cup (300 mL) thinly sliced carrots**

**water, to cover**

**1/3 cup (75 mL) butter**

**1/3 cup (75 mL) diced onion**

**1/3 cup (75 mL) gluten-free all-purpose flour (see page 9)**

**1/4 tsp (1 mL) celery seed**

**1/2 tsp (2 mL) salt**

**1/4 tsp (1 mL) pepper**

**1 3/4 cups (425 mL) chicken broth**

**1/3 cup (75 mL) half-and-half cream**

**1/3 cup (75 mL) milk**

Preheat oven to 425°F (220°C). Roll out 1 portion of pastry to about 1/8 inch (3 mm) thickness and line a 9 inch (23 cm) pie plate, or press directly into pie plate.

Place chicken, peas and carrots in a medium pot. Cover with water. Bring to a boil. Cook for 12 to 15 minutes, stirring occasionally, until carrots are softened. Drain. Spread mixture into pie crust.

Melt butter in a separate medium pot on medium. Add onion. Cook for about 5 minutes, stirring often, until softened. Add next 4 ingredients. Heat and stir for 30 seconds.

Slowly add next 3 ingredients to pot, one at a time. Stir on medium until boiling and thickened. Remove from heat. Spread over chicken in pie crust. Roll out second portion of dough to about 1/8 inch (3 mm) thickness. Cover pie with pastry. Trim dough and crimp decorative edge to seal. Cut several small slits in top pie crust. Bake on middle rack of preheated oven for 30 to 35 minutes until pastry is golden and filling is bubbling. Remove from oven and let stand on wire rack to cool for 10 to 12 minutes before serving.

*1 serving:* 1351 Calories; 65 g Total Fat (5 g Mono, 1 g Poly, 29 g Sat); 164 mg Cholesterol; 153 g Carbohydrate; 12 g Fibre; 38 g Protein; 1267 mg Sodium

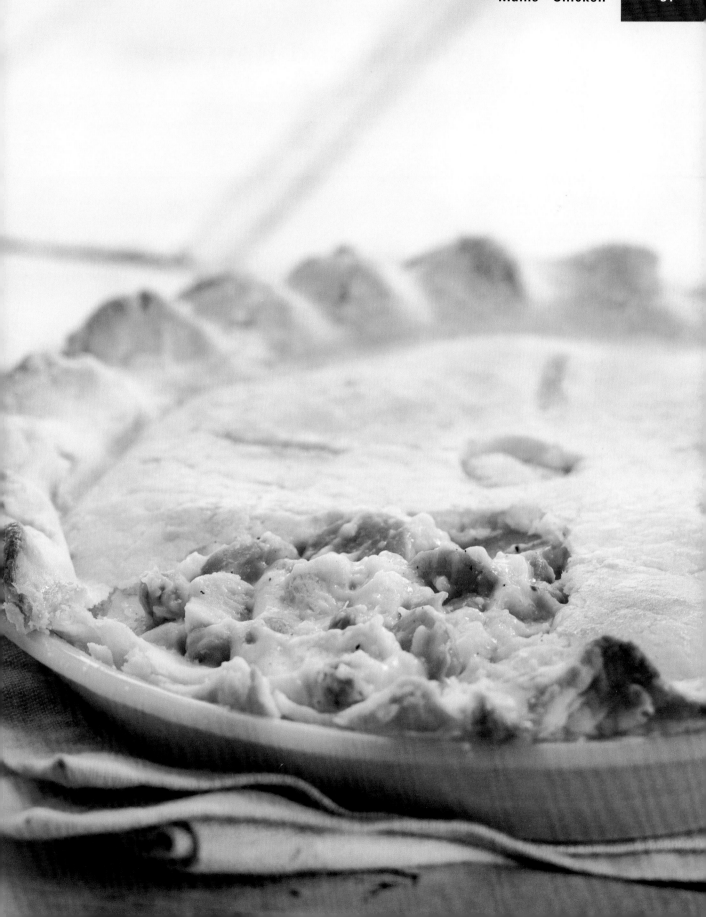

# Tortellini and Ravioli

## Serves 6

These small pasta pouches filled with cheese or meat require some extra work and preparation. But they are a nice addition to any gluten-free fare and are well worth it!

## Filling

1 1/2 cups (375 mL) lean ground chicken

1/2 cup (125 mL) cooked chopped spinach

3 slices prosciutto (or deli) ham

1/4 cup (60 mL) grated Parmesan cheese

1 large egg

1/2 tsp (2 mL) salt

1/8 tsp (0.5 mL) pepper

dash of ground nutmeg

chicken broth (optional)

## Pasta

1 cup (250 mL) yellow corn flour

1/4 cup (60 mL) pea starch

1 to 2 Tbsp (15 to 30 mL) pea fibre 80

1/4 cup (60 mL) rice flour

2 tsp (10 mL) xanthan gum

1 tsp (5 mL) fine sea salt

1 tsp (5 mL) guar gum

2 large eggs, room temperature

4 egg yolks (large), room temperature

(continued on next page)

**Filling:** Scramble-fry ground chicken in large frying pan on medium-high until no longer pink. Remove from heat.

Process spinach and next 6 ingredients in food processor until finely chopped but not paste-like. If mixture is too dry, add a bit of chicken broth. Add mixture to chicken and mix well. Set aside.

**Pasta:** Mix first 7 ingredients in a heavy-duty mixer.

Add eggs and egg yolks. Mix on medium with a paddle attachment for 2 to 3 minutes until well blended. Dough will feel pliable but not too soft.

If you're using a pasta machine, follow the manufacturer's instructions, understanding that gluten-free dough will be slightly stickier and less pliable. I roll the dough out to about 1/2 inch (12 mm) thickness between pieces of parchment paper before running through the pasta machine. Use a bit of pea starch for dusting if necessary to prevent sticking.

If you're not using a pasta machine, divide dough into small pieces about 1 1/2 to 2 inches (4 to 5 cm), or the size of a ping-pong ball. Lightly dust surface with pea starch. Roll out each piece as thin as possible.

For tortellini, you can use a pasta board, following manufacturer's instructions, or cut rolled-out dough into circles with 2 to 3 inch (5 to 7.5 cm) round cookie cutter. Add 1 1/2 tsp (7 mL) filling to each circle.

*(continued on next page)*

**Egg Wash:** Combine egg and milk or water in a small bowl. Brush pasta edges with egg wash. Roll pieces and pinch to seal. Bend sealed edge corners into the middle.

Pour water and salt into a large saucepan or Dutch oven. Bring to a boil. Cook tortellini, in batches, for about 5 minutes per batch until pasta is *al dente* and heated through. Filled pasta may need to be cooked a bit longer, about 12–14 minutes.

*1 serving: 321 Calories; 13 g Total Fat (3 g Mono, 1 g Poly, 4 g Sat); 346 mg Cholesterol; 28 g Carbohydrate; 4 g Fibre; 24 g Protein; 889 mg Sodium*

**Beef Stuffed Ravioli:** To make the filling for a smaller filled pasta variety, scramble-fry 1/2 lb (225 g) lean ground beef, 1 Tbsp (15 mL) butter and 1 minced garlic clove. Add 1/2 cup (125 mL) cooked chopped spinach, 2 eggs, 2 Tbsp (30 mL) grated Romano cheese, 1 Tbsp (15 mL) chopped fresh parsley and 1/8 tsp (0.5 mL) ground nutmeg. Use pasta recipe and directions given above for tortellini, but cut into 2 inch (5 cm) squares (half of squares will be ravioli bottoms and half will be tops). Follow directions above for egg wash and cooking.

**Egg Wash**

1 large egg, fork-beaten

1/2 tsp (2 mL) milk or water

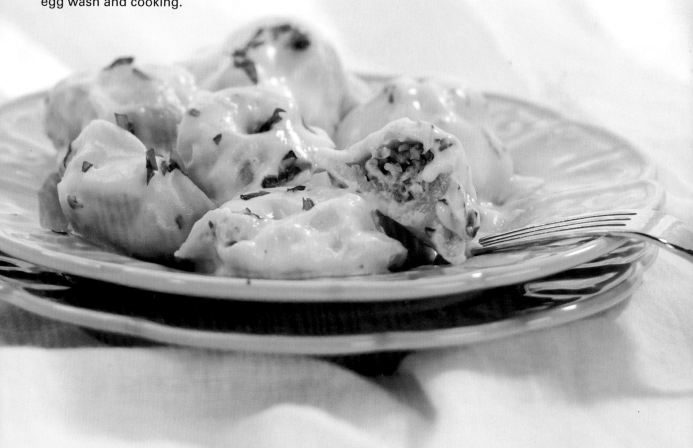

# Thanksgiving Turkey Dinner

## Serves 8 to 10

Probably one of our most-loved traditions is the annual Thanksgiving dinner with friends and family. What a wonderful time to enjoy each other's company and share great food. This turkey recipe offers a little twist to the usual seasoning. Oven-baked sweet potatoes and other side dishes round out this lovely meal.

## Turkey

1 1/2 Tbsp (25 mL) egg, fork-beaten (about 1/3 of an egg)

1/4 cup (60 mL) canola oil

1 1/2 tsp (7 mL) white vinegar

1/8 tsp (0.5 mL) dry mustard powder

1/8 tsp (0.5 mL) salt

2 to 3 x 12 oz (341 mL) bottles gluten-free beer (such as Bard's)

1/2 cup (125 mL) butter, softened

12 to 18 lb (5.4 to 8.2 kg) whole turkey, thawed if frozen

Poultry Stuffing (see page 148), double or triple the recipe depending on the bird size

## Gravy

3 to 4 Tbsp (45 to 60 mL) gluten-free all-purpose flour (see page 9)

1 1/4 cups (300 mL) milk

1 1/4 cups (300 mL) water

1/2 to 1 tsp (2 to 5 mL) salt

1/8 to 1/4 tsp (0.5 to 1 mL) pepper

(continued on next page)

**Turkey:** Preheat oven to 325°F (160°C). Whisk first 5 ingredients in a small bowl until a cream-like consistency is formed.

Combine beer and butter in a separate small bowl.

Loosely fill body cavity of turkey with stuffing. Secure cavity with wooden picks or small metal skewers. Tie wings close to body with butcher's string. Tie legs to tail. Transfer turkey to a deep roasting pan. Pour beer mixture over turkey. Spread canola oil mixture over turkey. Cover roasting pan with foil. Bake for 4 hours, basting turkey occasionally with pan juices. Remove foil. Bake, uncovered, for 1/2 to 1 1/2 hours until meat thermometer inserted in thickest part of thigh reaches 180°F (82°C). Temperature of stuffing should reach at least 165°F (74°C). Transfer turkey to a large cutting board. Drain and discard all but 1/3 cup (75 mL) drippings. Remove and discard string and skewers. Cover turkey with foil. Let stand for 30 to 35 minutes before carving. You can remove the stuffing, or serve it with the turkey on a platter.

**Gravy:** Heat reserved drippings in same pan on medium. Add flour. Heat and stir for 1 minute. Slow add milk and water, stirring constantly with a whisk or fork and scraping any brown bits from bottom of pan. Cook on medium to high for 3 to 5 minutes, stirring constantly, until gravy is thickened. Add salt and pepper to taste.

(continued on next page)

**Sweet Potatoes:** Spread sweet potato slices evenly onto greased baking sheet. Mix butter and brown sugar. Brush on top of sweet potato. Bake in a 325°F (160°C) oven for 40 minutes until softened.

**Brussels Sprouts:** Melt butter in a large saucepan on medium. Add Brussels sprouts. Cook for 5 to 10 minutes, stirring occasionally. Add remaining 4 ingredients. Bring to a boil. Cook for about 10 minutes until sprouts are desired crispness. Discard lemon peel before serving.

*1 serving:* 2038 Calories; 110 g Total Fat (19 g Mono, 5 g Poly, 42 g Sat); 604 mg Cholesterol; 109 g Carbohydrate; 10 g Fibre; 150 g Protein; 1711 mg Sodium

## Sweet Potatoes

3 medium orange-fleshed sweet potatoes, thinly sliced

1/2 cup (125 mL) butter, melted

1/2 cup (125 mL) brown sugar

## Brussels Sprouts

1/2 cup (125 mL) butter

2 lbs (900 kg) Brussels sprouts

1 cup (250 mL) chicken broth

yellow peel from 2 lemon slices (not inner white pith)

1 tsp (5 mL) salt

1/2 tsp (2 mL) fresh marjoram

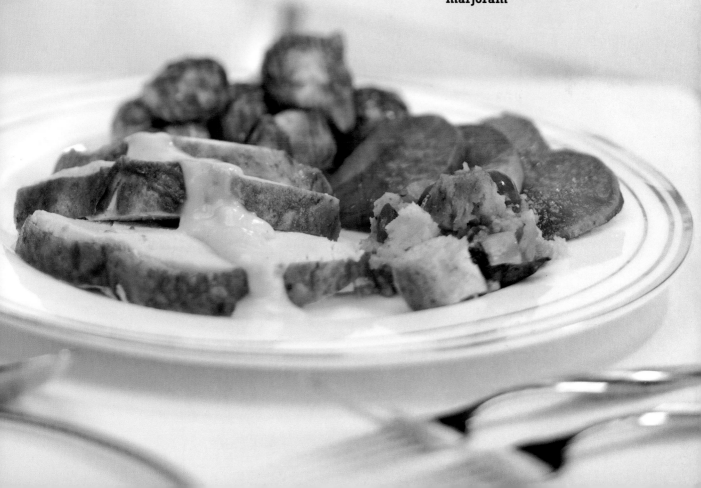

# Creamy Turkey Casserole

## Serves 8

The morning after your festive Thanksgiving dinner begs the question: how do you use up any leftover turkey? This creamy casserole will please everyone's tastebuds.

1/3 cup (75 mL) butter, melted

2 to 3 cups (500 to 750 mL) chopped cooked turkey

2 large sweet potatoes, diced

3 cups (750 mL) chopped broccoli florets

6 Tbsp (90 mL) all-purpose gluten-free flour (see page 9)

2 cups (500 mL) half-and-half cream

2 cups (500 mL) milk

1 cup (250 mL) grated Cheddar cheese

1 cup (250 mL) grated mozzarella cheese

2 garlic cloves, minced

2 tsp (10 mL) salt

dash of cayenne pepper

1/3 cup (75 mL) grated Parmesan cheese

Preheat oven to 400°F (200°C). Grease a 9 x 13 inch (23 x 33 cm) baking pan. Combine first 4 ingredients in a large bowl.

Combine next 8 ingredients in a separate bowl. Layer ingredients in prepared pan as follows:

- 1/3 turkey mixture
- 1/3 cheese mixture
- 1/3 turkey mixture
- 1/3 cheese mixture
- 1/3 turkey mixture
- 1/3 cheese mixture

Top with Parmesan cheese. Bake in oven for about 40 minutes until sweet potatoes are softened. Broil for 1 to 2 minutes to brown top if desired.

*1 serving: 417 Calories; 26 g Total Fat (7 g Mono, 1 g Poly, 16 g Sat); 100 mg Cholesterol; 22 g Carbohydrate; 2 g Fibre; 24 g Protein; 1310 mg Sodium*

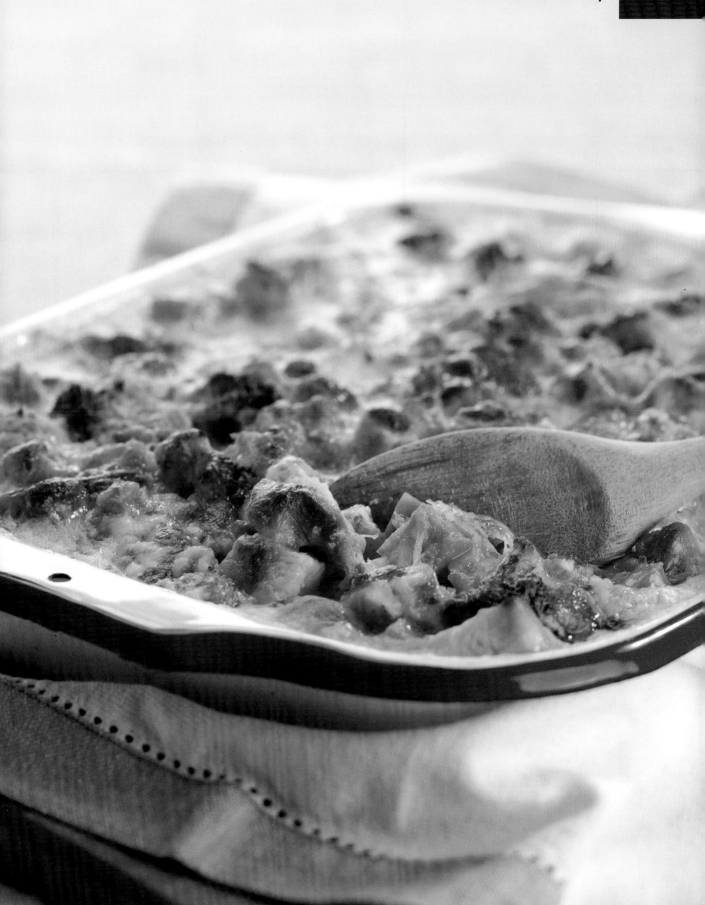

# Fish Sticks

## Makes 16

Slim breaded pieces of fish, oven-baked with a hint of spice. Eat the fish sticks by themselves or as an addition to any meal. Serve with a gluten-free dipping sauce, such as plum sauce or a creamy dressing.

**2 cups (500 mL) gluten-free panko crumbs**

**1 tsp (5 mL) salt**

**1/4 tsp (1 mL) cayenne pepper**

**1/8 tsp (0.5 mL) pepper**

**2 large eggs, fork-beaten**

**1 1/2 to 2 lbs (680 to 900 g) medium boneless cod fillets, cut into 3/4 x 3 inch (2 x 7.5 cm) strips**

**3 Tbsp (45 mL) cooking oil**

Preheat oven to 450°F (230°C). Combine first 4 ingredients in a shallow dish. Place eggs in separate shallow dish.

Press cod pieces in panko mixture. Dip in egg. Press cod pieces into panko mixture again until coated. Discard any remaining panko mixture and egg.

Place a baking pan in preheated oven for 30 seconds. Remove from oven and add oil, spreading evenly over bottom. Place fish sticks in baking pan. Bake for 10 to 12 minutes in oven, flipping at halftime, until fish flakes easily when tested with a fork.

*1 stick:* 256 Calories; 4 g Total Fat (2 g Mono, 1 g Poly, 1 g Sat); 174 mg Cholesterol; 5 g Carbohydrate; 0 g Fibre; 48 g Protein; 469 mg Sodium

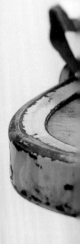

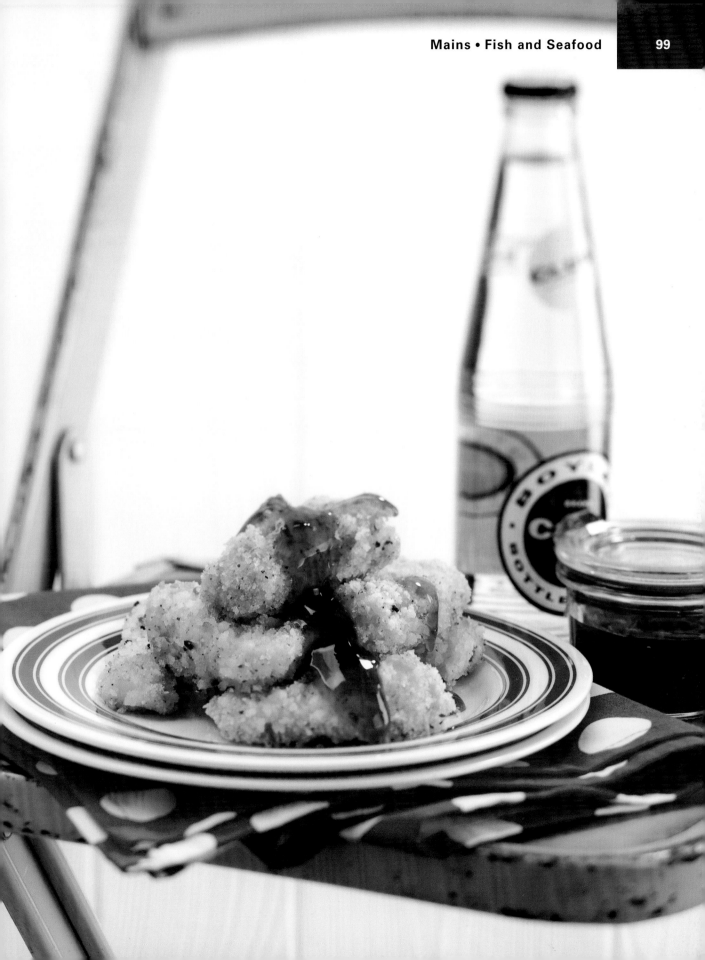

# Fish and Chips

## Serves 6

A soft white fish in a tasty batter served with fries—classic pub food. Serve your fish and chips with salt and vinegar, or with tartar sauce.

## Chips

**lard, for frying**

**6 large potatoes, cut into sticks or wedges**

## Batter

**1 cup (250 mL) white rice flour**

**1/2 cup (125 mL) pea starch**

**1/4 cup (60 mL) tapioca starch**

**1/4 cup (60 mL) yellow corn flour**

**2 Tbsp (30 mL) sugar**

**1 Tbsp (15 mL) paprika**

**1 Tbsp (15 mL) xanthan gum**

**2 tsp (10 mL) baking powder**

**1 tsp (5 mL) pepper**

**1/2 tsp (2 mL) salt**

**1 cup (250 mL) milk (or almond milk)**

**1/2 cup (125 mL) gluten-free beer (such as Bards)**

*(continued on next page)*

**Chips:** Heat lard in deep fryer to 350°F (175°C) according to manufacturer's instructions. Deep-fry potato pieces, in batches, in hot cooking oil for 2 1/2 to 3 minutes until golden brown. Remove each batch to paper towels to drain. Cover to keep warm. Set aside.

**Batter:** Mix next 10 ingredients in a large bowl.

Mix remaining 6 ingredients in a separate bowl. Add egg mixture to flour mixture. Mix until a smooth batter is formed.

Dip fish in batter to cover. Drop into preheated deep-fryer oil. Turn pieces when they rise to the surface. Deep fry for 2 1/2 to 3 minutes until golden brown. Remove to paper towels to drain. Keep warm in a 175°F (80°C) oven.

Deep-fry potato pieces again for 30 to 60 seconds before serving.

*1 serving: 935 Calories; 36 g Total Fat (7 g Mono, 3 g Poly, 11 g Sat); 247 mg Cholesterol; 114 g Carbohydrate; 9 g Fibre; 38 g Protein; 459 mg Sodium*

4 egg yolks (large)

1 large egg

1/4 cup (60 mL) cooking oil

2 tsp (10 mL) vanilla

1 1/2 to 2 lbs (680 to 900 g)
medium tilapia or cod
fillets, cut into 2- to 3-inch
(5 to 7.5 cm) slices

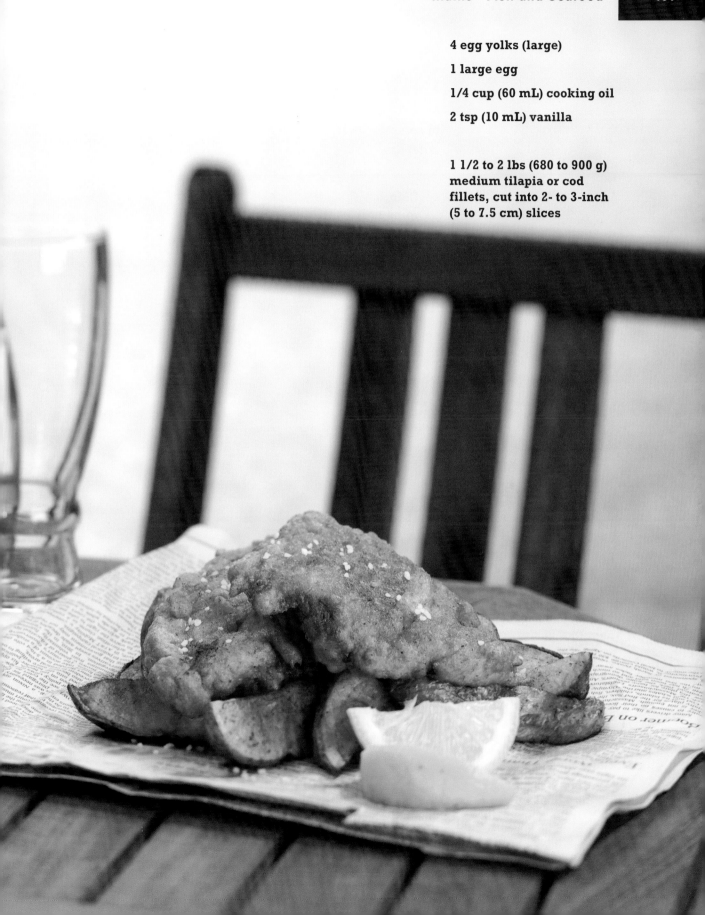

# Curry Cream Shrimp

## Serves 6

A creamy, well-spiced shrimp main course, satisfying and pleasing to the senses. Served over pasta.

**6 Tbsp (90 mL) butter**

**2 1/2 cups (625 mL) finely chopped onion**

**2 tsp (10 mL) curry powder**

**6 to 8 Tbsp (90 to 120 mL) gluten-free all-purpose flour (see page 9)**

**7 Tbsp (105 mL) tomato paste**

**2 cups (500 mL) water**

**3 cups (750 mL) whipping cream**

**1 1/2 tsp (7 mL) salt**

**1 tsp (5 mL) pepper**

**1/2 tsp (2 mL) cayenne pepper**

**4 1/2 to 5 lbs (2 to 2.3 kg) uncooked medium shrimp (peeled and de-veined)**

**12 oz (340 g) gluten-free pasta**

**3 to 5 Tbsp (45 to 75 mL) chopped fresh parsley**

Heat butter in a large pot on medium. Add onion. Cook for 5 to 10 minutes, stirring often, until softened. Add curry powder. Cook for 30 seconds. Add flour slowly, stirring until well mixed.

Slowly add tomato paste, water and whipping cream, stirring constantly. Bring to a boil for 2 to 3 minutes. Add next 3 ingredients. Cook for 30 seconds. Reduce heat to medium.

Add shrimp. Cook for 3 to 4 minutes until shrimp are pink. Remove from heat. Cover to keep warm.

Prepare pasta according to package directions. Drain. Place pasta on individual plates and top with curried shrimp. Garnish with parsley.

*1 serving:* 1092 Calories; 57 g Total Fat (14 g Mono, 2 g Poly, 31 g Sat); 680 mg Cholesterol; 69 g Carbohydrate; 4 g Fibre; 78 g Protein; 1290 mg Sodium

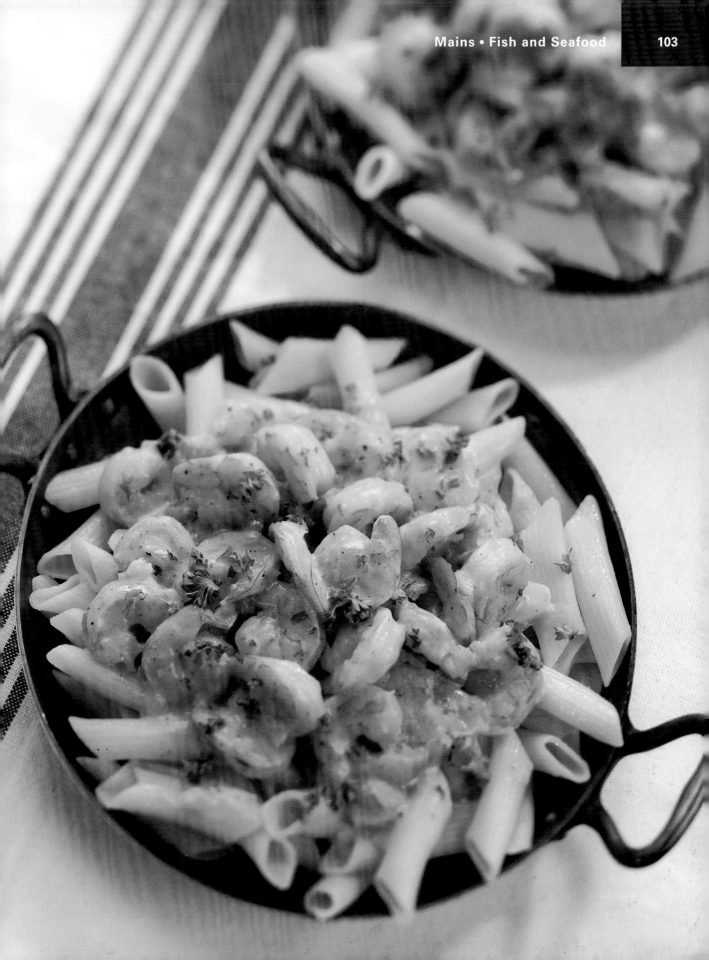

# Slow Sweet and Spicy Seafood Stew

## Serves 6 to 8

A lazy stew that's cooked in your slow cooker. The combination of spices and subtle sweetness fills your kitchen with a tantalizing aroma. Make sure not to add the seafood too early.

**2 lbs (900 g) potatoes, peeled and diced**

**1 lb (454 g) yellow turnip (rutabaga), peeled and diced**

**1 lb (454 g) sliced carrots**

**3 cups (750 mL) tomato sauce**

**1/4 cup (60 mL) ketchup**

**2 Tbsp (30 mL) honey**

**1 Tbsp (15 mL) Dijon mustard**

**1 Tbsp (15 mL) molasses**

**2 tsp (10 mL) Italian seasoning**

**1 1/2 tsp (7 mL) minced garlic**

**1 1/2 tsp (7 mL) turmeric**

**1 tsp (5 mL) cayenne pepper**

**3/4 tsp (4 mL) salt**

**1 1/2 cups (375 mL) water**

**1 lb (454 g) large sea scallops**

**1 lb (454 g) uncooked medium shrimp (peeled and de-veined)**

**2 to 3 Tbsp (30 to 45 mL) cornstarch (optional)**

Combine first 13 ingredients in a 5 to 6 quart (5 to 6 L) slow cooker. Cook, covered, on Low for 5 hours or on High for 3 to 4 hours.

Add water, scallops and shrimp. Add cornstarch if a thicker consistency is desired. Stir. Cook, covered, for 15 to 20 minutes on High until shrimp are pink.

*1 serving*: 392 Calories; 2 g Total Fat (0 g Mono, 1 g Poly, 0 g Sat); 140 mg Cholesterol; 60 g Carbohydrate; 7 g Fibre; 34 g Protein; 1523 mg Sodium

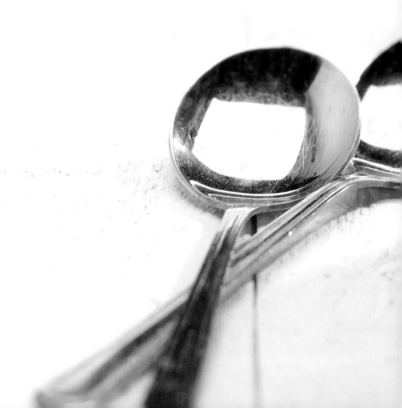

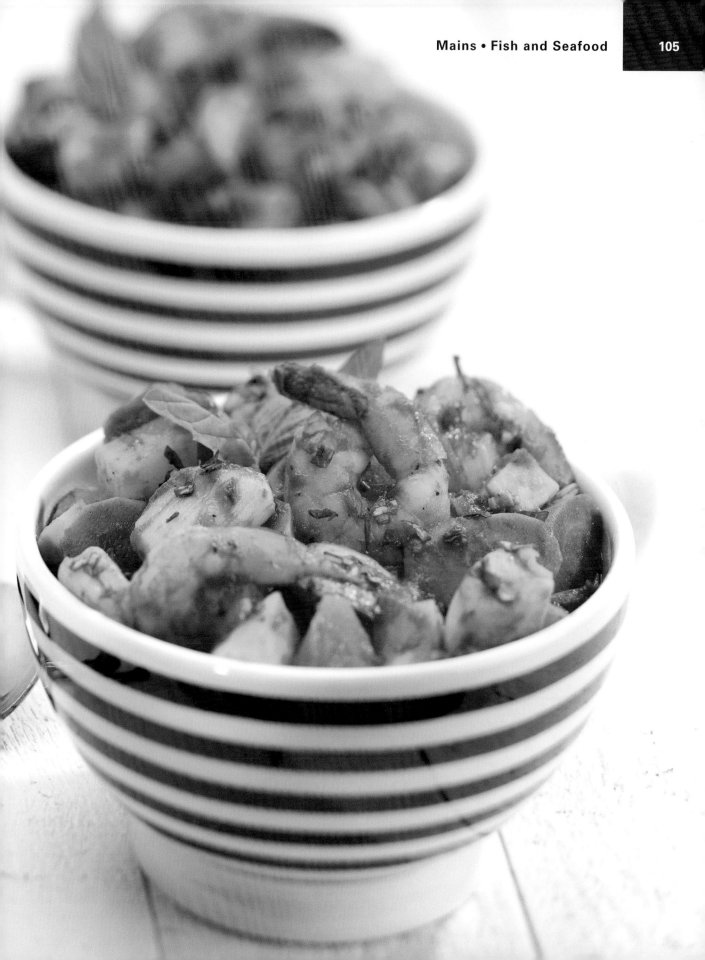

# Breaded Pan-fried Trout

## Serves 4

A very simple pan-fried dish. You can substitute your favourite type of fish for the trout. You can also premix the dry ingredients and take them with you on your next fishing trip—then enjoy your catch right over the campfire! Serve with rice and broccoli for a perfect meal.

**4 x 1 to 1 1/2 lbs (454 to 680 g) trout fillets, skin and any small bones removed**

Rinse trout and pat dry.

Combine next 4 ingredients in a large resealable bag. Add fillets, 1 piece at a time. Toss until coated.

**1 cup (250 mL) cornmeal**

**2 Tbsp (30 mL) all-purpose gluten-free flour (see page 9)**

**1/8 tsp (0.5 mL) salt**

**1/8 tsp (0.5 mL) pepper**

Melt butter in a large frying pan on medium. Add fillets. Cook for 4 to 5 minutes per side until fish flakes easily when tested with a fork. Serve with Béchamel sauce.

**6 Tbsp (90 mL) butter**

**2 to 3 cups (500 to 750 mL) Béchamel sauce (see page 154)**

*1 serving*: 634 Calories; 31 g Total Fat (8 g Mono, 3 g Poly, 17 g Sat); 162 mg Cholesterol; 46 g Carbohydrate; 1 g Fibre; 39 g Protein; 404 mg Sodium

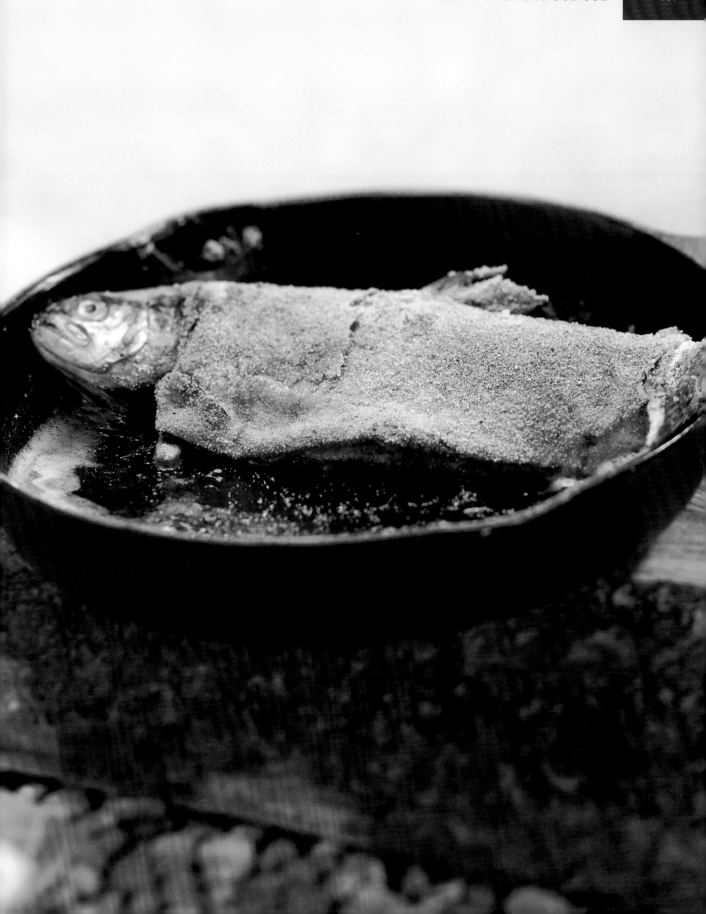

# Scallops and Shrimp Pasta

## Serves 6 to 8

An easy pasta and seafood meal with a wine and cream sauce. It tastes wonderful and looks very pretty, with a topping of tomatoes, herbs and cheese added at the end.

**2 x 12 oz (340 g) packages gluten-free linguine or fettucine**

**1/2 cup (125 mL) olive oil**

**1 medium red onion, sliced into rings**

**3/4 lb (340 g) large sea scallops**

**3/4 lb (340 g) uncooked shrimp (peeled and de-veined)**

**1 1/2 cups (375 mL) white wine**

**1 1/2 cups (375 mL) sliced smoked salmon, cut into 1/2 inch (12 mm) strips**

**3 cups (750 mL) whipping cream**

**1 1/2 Tbsp (25 mL) minced garlic**

**1 cup (250 mL) grated Parmesan cheese**

**1 1/2 tsp (7 mL) salt**

**3/4 tsp (4 mL) pepper**

Cook pasta according to package directions. Drain. Return to same pot. Cover to keep warm.

Heat oil in a large frying pan on medium. Add onions. Cook for about 5 minutes until softened.

Add next 3 ingredients. Cook for about 3 minutes until shrimp just start to turn pink.

Add next 6 ingredients. Cook for about 3 minutes, stirring occasionally. Remove from heat. Add pasta. Stir until well mixed. Let stand for 2 to 3 minutes.

Top with remaining 4 ingredients just before serving.

*1 serving:* 1198 Calories; 68 g Total Fat (27 g Mono, 4 g Poly, 30 g Sat); 266 mg Cholesterol; 97 g Carbohydrate; 11 g Fibre; 45 g Protein; 1373 mg Sodium

*(continued on next page)*

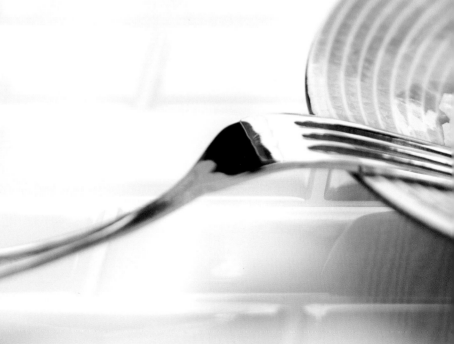

2 medium Roma tomatoes, chopped

1 to 2 Tbsp (15 to 30 mL) chopped fresh parsley

1 to 2 Tbsp (15 to 30 mL) fresh basil, cut into strips

1 to 2 Tbsp (15 to 30 mL) grated Parmesan cheese

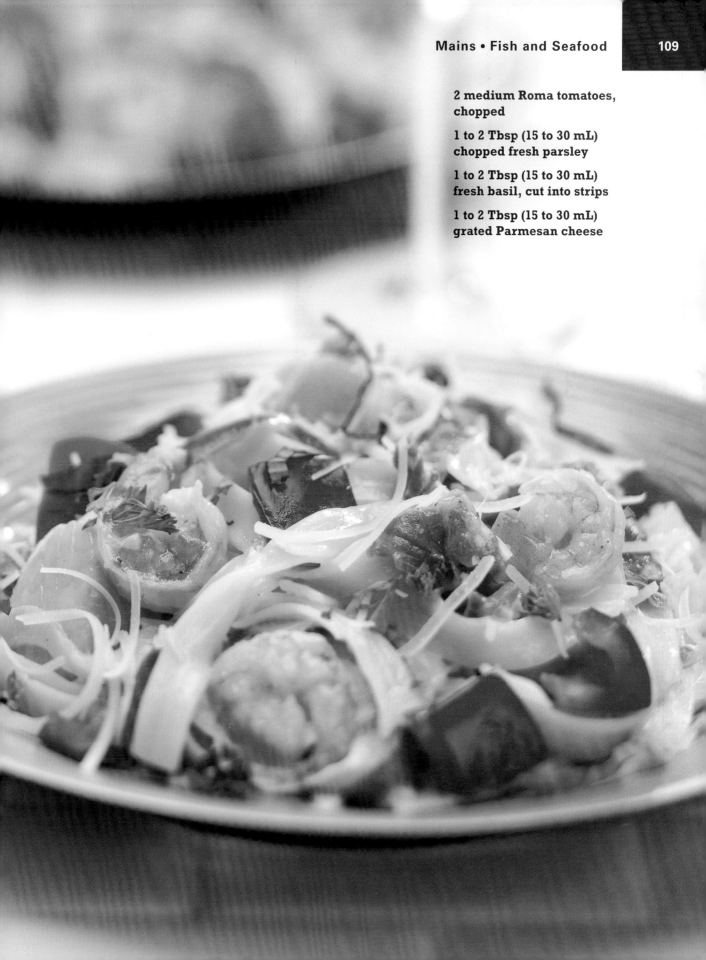

# Asian Pork Stew

## Serves 6

Sweet and sour notes combine with colourful vegetables and pork for a fast and satisfying meal.

**3 Tbsp (45 mL) cooking oil**

**3/4 tsp (4 mL) anise seed**

**1/2 tsp (2 mL) fennel seed**

**1/2 tsp (2 mL) ground cinnamon**

**1/2 tsp (2 mL) ground cloves**

**1/2 tsp (2 mL) pepper**

**2 lbs (900 g) boneless centre-cut pork chops, cut into 1 1/2 inch (4 cm) cubes**

**3 Tbsp (45 mL) gluten-free all-purpose flour (see page 9)**

**3 to 4 celery stalks, sliced**

**3/4 cup (175 mL) sliced green onions**

**1/2 to 1 lb (225 to 454 g) fresh white mushrooms, sliced**

**1 1/2 cups (375 mL) chicken broth**

**2 Tbsp (30 mL) gluten-free tamari sauce**

**2 Tbsp (30 mL) gluten-free teriyaki sauce (see page 156)**

**1 Tbsp (15 mL) rice vinegar**

**1 Tbsp (15 mL) honey**

**3/4 tsp (4 mL) ground ginger**

Heat oil in a large frying pan or stock pot. Add next 5 ingredients. Stir and heat for 1 minute.

Add pork. Cook for 2 to 3 minutes, stirring occasionally, until browned on all sides. Sprinkle with flour. Stir.

Add next 9 ingredients. Stir. Cook, covered, for 30 minutes.

Add green beans. Cook for 10 to 15 minutes until beans are tender. If a thicker consistency is desired, add cornstarch. Cook, stirring occasionally, for about 3 minutes until thickened.

Sprinkle individual servings with sesame seeds.

*1 serving: 480 Calories; 23 g Total Fat (11 g Mono, 4 g Poly, 6 g Sat); 138 mg Cholesterol; 15 g Carbohydrate; 3 g Fibre; 52 g Protein; 624 mg Sodium*

*(continued on next page)*

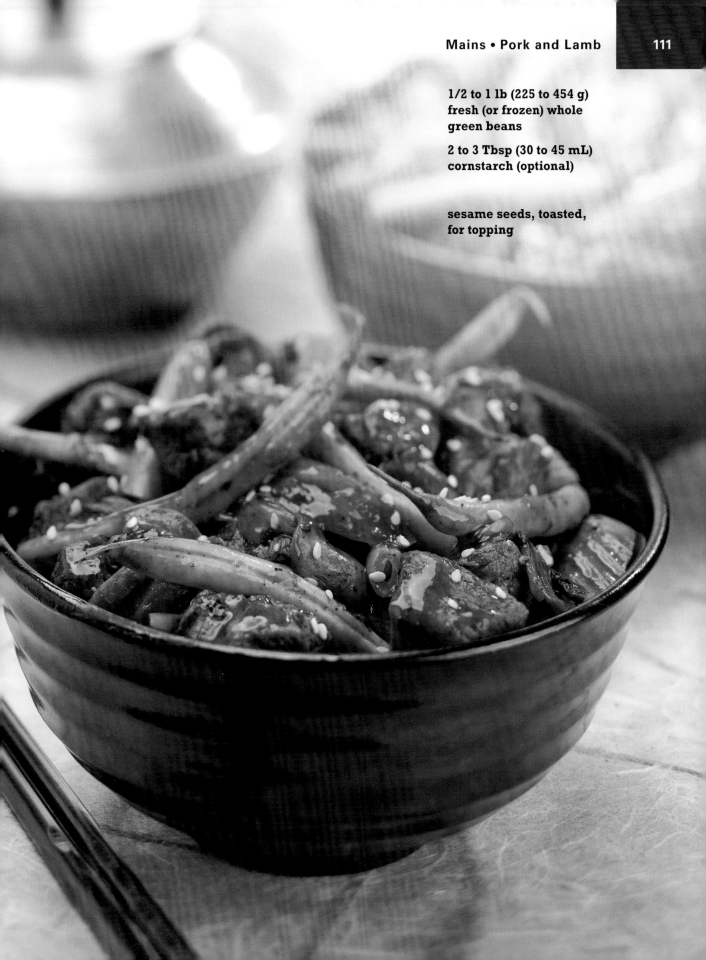

1/2 to 1 lb (225 to 454 g)
fresh (or frozen) whole
green beans

2 to 3 Tbsp (30 to 45 mL)
cornstarch (optional)


sesame seeds, toasted,
for topping

# Wiener Schnitzel

## Serves 6 to 8

Not to be confused with hot dogs or the famous dachshund! This wiener schnitzel recipe is a thin, tenderized, breaded pork steak, although traditionally the dish was made from veal. Try serving with fries and applesauce.

**2 cups (500 mL) gluten-free bread crumbs (see page 9) or panko crumbs**

**grated zest from 2 lemons**

**1 Tbsp (15 mL) paprika**

**1 tsp (5 mL) salt**

**1 tsp (5 mL) pepper**

**1/2 to 1 cup (125 to 250 mL) sweet rice flour**

**2 large eggs, fork-beaten**

**6 to 8 thin pork (or veal) steaks**

**1/2 to 1 cup (125 to 250 mL) lard or cooking oil**

Combine first 5 ingredients in a shallow dish. Place flour in a small bowl. Place eggs in shallow dish.

Place pork steaks between 2 sheets of plastic wrap. Pound with mallet or rolling pin to 1/4 inch (6 mm) thickness. Press both sides of pork into flour. Dip into egg. Press both sides in crumb mixture until coated. Discard any remaining flour, egg and crumb mixture.

Melt lard to about 1/4 inch (6 mm) up sides of frying pan. Heat on medium-high. Cook pork for 3 to 5 minutes per side until fully cooked and golden brown.

*1 serving:* 427 Calories; 26 g Total Fat (14 g Mono, 6 g Poly, 4 g Sat); 119 mg Cholesterol; 23 g Carbohydrate; 2 g Fibre; 24 g Protein; 483 mg Sodium

(continued on next page)

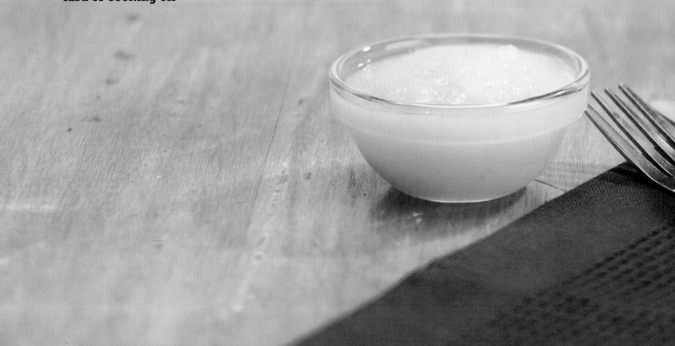

**Breaded Pork Chops:** Replace lemon zest with
2 tsp (10 mL) Italian seasoning. Replace pork steaks
with pork chops. Do not pound.

**Breaded Sole:** Replace pork with 6 to 8 medium
sole fillets. Do not pound. Cook breaded fillets for about
6 minutes per side until fish flakes easily when tested with
a fork.

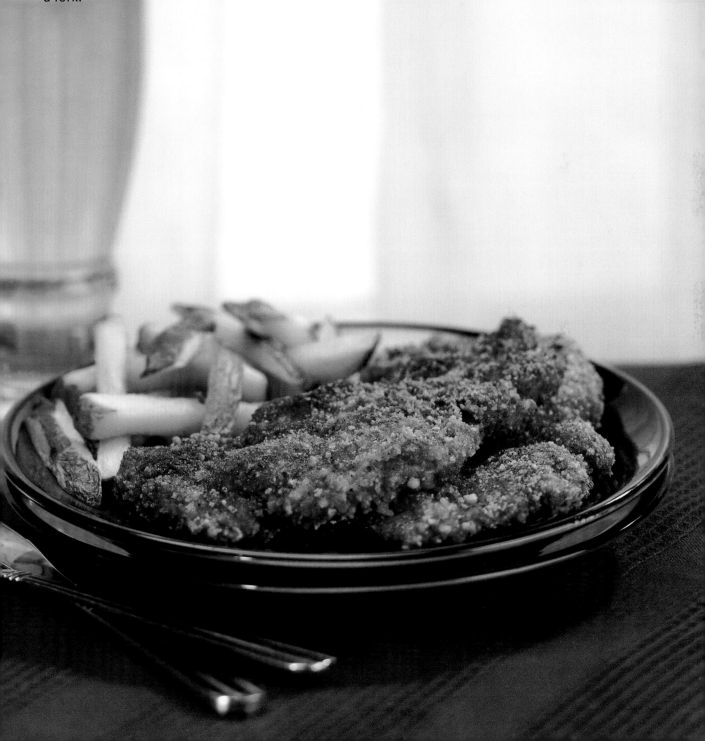

# Sweet and Sour Pork

## Serves 6 to 8

These little fried dough balls with pork are served with vegetables and rice, all covered with a delicious sweet and sour sauce.

lard, for frying

### Batter

1 cup (250 mL) white rice flour

1/2 cup (125 mL) pea starch

1/4 cup (60 mL) tapioca starch

1/4 cup (60 mL) yellow corn flour

2 Tbsp (30 mL) sugar

1 Tbsp (15 mL) paprika

1 Tbsp (15 mL) xanthan gum

2 tsp (10 mL) baking powder

1/2 tsp (2 mL) salt

1 tsp (5 mL) pepper

1 1/2 cups (375 mL) milk (or almond milk)

4 egg yolks (large)

1 large egg

1/4 cup (60 mL) cooking oil

2 tsp (10 mL) vanilla extract

6 x 4 to 6 oz (113 to 170 g) medium boneless pork chops, cut into 1/2-inch (6 mm) cubes

Heat lard in deep fryer to 350°F (175°C) as per manufacturer's instructions.

**Batter:** Mix next 10 ingredients in a large bowl.

Mix next 5 ingredients in a separate bowl. Add egg mixture to flour mixture. Mix until a smooth batter is formed.

Dip pork cubes in batter to cover. Drop pork into preheated lard. Turn pieces when they rise to the surface. Deep-fry for about 3 minutes until brown. Remove to paper towels to drain. Cover or place in a 175°F (80°C) oven to keep warm.

**Sweet and Sour Sauce:** Combine first amount of chicken broth and cornstarch.

Combine next 6 ingredients in a small pot. Bring to a boil. Add cornstarch mixture. Heat and stir until thickened. Remove from heat. Cover to keep warm.

Prepare rice and vegetables according to package directions. Serve rice, vegetables and pork balls topped with sweet and sour sauce.

*1 serving:* 1079 Calories; 50 g Total Fat (14 g Mono, 5 g Poly, 15 g Sat); 263 mg Cholesterol; 121 g Carbohydrate; 9 g Fibre; 36 g Protein; 684 mg Sodium

### Sweet and Sour Chicken Balls: Omit pork. Replace with 6 x 4 to 6 oz (113 to 170 g) boneless, skinless chicken breast halves, cut into 1/4 inch (6 mm) cubes.

*(continued on next page)*

## Sweet and Sour Sauce

1/3 cup (75 mL) chicken broth

1 to 2 Tbsp (15 to 30 mL) cornstarch

1 1/4 cup (300 mL) chicken broth

2 Tbsp (30 mL) gluten-free plum sauce

2 Tbsp (30 mL) honey

1 1/2 Tbsp (25 mL) rice vinegar

1 to 2 Tbsp (15 to 30 mL) cornstarch

3/4 tsp (4 mL) ground ginger

3 cups (750 mL) fresh or frozen mixed stir-fry vegetables

2 cups (500 mL) rice

# Perogies

## Makes 28 perogies

Do you like potato and cheddar or onion and bacon, or are you more adventurous and fill your perogies with fruit fillings? Whichever way you like them, perogies are a great quick meal. Savoury perogy varieties are often served with sour cream, glazed onions and sausage. I like to make a whole bunch of perogies at a time and freeze the extras for another day.

## Dough

**2 large eggs, room temperature**

**1 3/4 cups (425 mL) gluten-free all-purpose flour (see page 9)**

**1/2 cup (125 mL) water, approximately**

**1 Tbsp (15 mL) sour cream**

**1/4 tsp (1 mL) xanthan gum**

## Filling

**3 medium potatoes, peeled, cooked, mashed and cooled**

**2 Tbsp (30 mL) butter, approximately**

**1 small onion, chopped**

**1 garlic clove, minced**

**1 cup (250 mL) cooked and crumbled bacon**

**19 cups (4.75 L) water**

**3 to 4 Tbsp (45 to 60 mL) butter**

**1/8 tsp (0.5 mL) salt**

**1/8 tsp (0.5 mL) pepper**

**Dough:** Beat eggs in a large bowl. Add next 4 ingredients. If dough is sticky, add more flour. Turn out dough onto surface lightly dusted with gluten-free flour. Roll out dough to desired thickness. Cut out circles with 2 inch (5 cm) round cookie cutter.

**Filling:** Mix first 5 ingredients together. Place 1 Tbsp (15 mL) filling on each dough circle. Fold in half. Press edges together with a wet fork to seal.

Pour water into a large saucepan or Dutch oven. Bring to a boil. Cook perogies in batches for 2 to 3 minutes, stirring occasionally, until perogies float to the top. Cook for 1 minute before removing with a slotted spoon to sieve. Drain. Cook in frying pan with butter until lightly browned. Add salt and pepper to taste.

*1 perogie: 79 Calories; 4 g Total Fat (1 g Mono, 0 g Poly, 2 g Sat); 24 mg Cholesterol; 9 g Carbohydrate; 1 g Fibre; 3 g Protein; 61 mg Sodium*

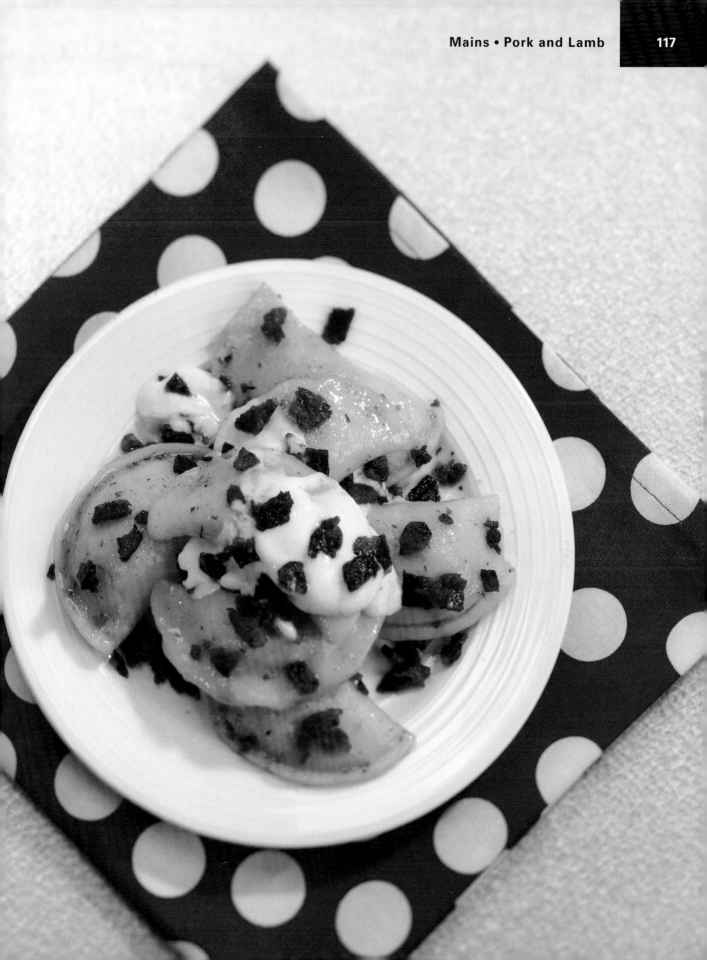

# Pizza Pockets

## Makes 12

These delicious pizza-dough pastries with a meaty tomato filling and stretchy cheese make the perfect handheld meal. Can be stored frozen for a quick lunchtime snack.

2/3 cup (150 mL) sweet rice flour

2/3 cup (150 mL) tapioca starch

1/3 cup (75 mL) pea starch

2 Tbsp (30 mL) sugar

2 Tbsp (30 mL) whey powder

1 1/2 Tbsp (25 mL) active dry yeast

1 1/2 Tbsp (25 mL) pea fibre III

2 tsp (10 mL) xanthan gum

1 1/4 tsp (6 mL) guar gum

1/4 tsp (1 mL) salt

1/2 cup (125 mL) water

3 Tbsp (45 mL) cooking oil

2 egg whites (large), room temperature

1 large egg, room temperature

(continued on next page)

Preheat oven to 400°F (200°C). Mix first 10 ingredients in a medium metal bowl.

Mix next 4 ingredients in a separate bowl. Add egg mixture to flour mixture. Knead together or use a heavy-duty mixer with a dough hook attachment.

Turn out dough onto surface lightly dusted with sweet rice flour. Divide dough into 2 balls. Roll dough pieces out to desired thickness.

For round pizza pockets, cut 24 circles with a 3-inch (7.5 cm) round cookie cutter (12 for the top and 12 for the bottom). For half moon–shaped pizza pockets, cut dough into 12 larger circles, using one piece for each pocket by folding one side over the other.

**Filling:** Mix ham and cheese. Spread 1 tsp (5 mL) pizza sauce onto 12 dough pieces. Place two pepperoni pieces in centre. Divide ham and cheese mixture evenly over pepperoni. Top with 1/2 to 1 tsp (2 to 5 mL) pizza sauce. Cover with remaining dough slices or fold pieces over. Press edges together with a wet fork to seal.

(continued on next page)

**Egg Wash:** Combine egg and milk or water in a small bowl. Brush pizza pockets with egg wash. Bake on greased baking sheets in preheated oven for 20 to 25 minutes until golden brown.

*1 pocket: 171 Calories; 7 g Total Fat (4 g Mono, 1 g Poly, 2 g Sat); 48 mg Cholesterol; 20 g Carbohydrate; 2 g Fibre; 7 g Protein; 308 mg Sodium*

## Filling

1/2 cup (125 mL) deli ham, finely cubed

3/4 to 1 cup (175 to 250 mL) grated mozzarella cheese

7 1/2 oz (213 mL) gluten-free pizza sauce

10 to 12 slices pizza pepperoni, cut in half

## Egg Wash

1 large egg, fork-beaten

1/2 tsp (2 mL) milk or water

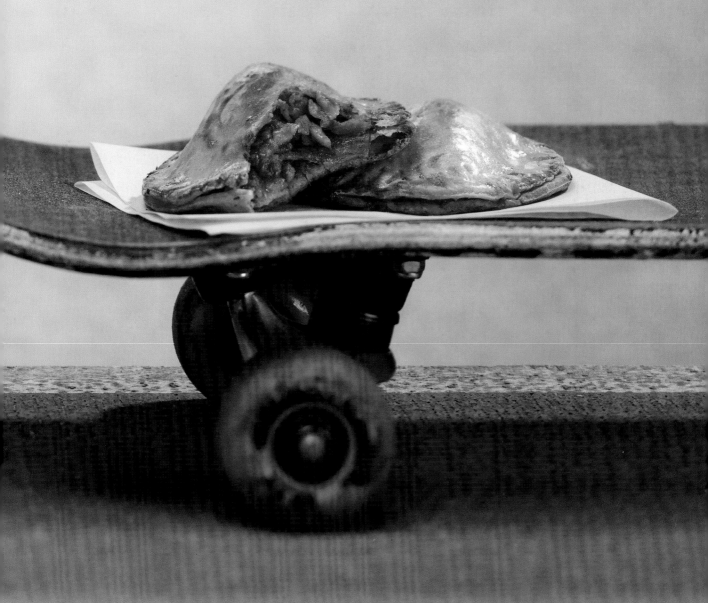

# Quiche Lorraine

## Serves 6

A rich combination of cream, eggs, cheese and bacon makes for a tasty open-faced pie. This recipe makes two 9-inch (23 cm) pies. This dish can be frozen. You can use premade gluten-free pie crusts or make the pastry recipe below.

## Pastry Crust

1 cup (250 mL) white rice flour

1/2 cup (125 mL) sweet rice flour

1/2 cup (125 mL) tapioca starch

1/4 cup (60 mL) pea starch

1 Tbsp (15 mL) pea fibre 80

1 Tbsp (15 mL) sugar

1 1/2 tsp (7 mL) xanthan gum

1 tsp (5 mL) baking powder

1 tsp (5 mL) salt

3/4 cup (175 mL) lard


1 large egg

2 Tbsp (30 mL) vinegar

2 Tbsp (30 mL) water, approximately

*(continued on next page)*

**Pastry Crust:** Preheat oven to 450°F (230°C). Combine first 9 ingredients in a large bowl. Cut in lard until mixture resembles coarse crumbs.

Add egg, vinegar and water, if necessary (only add water if dough is too dry to make a pliable pie dough). Blend until mixture starts to come together. Do not over mix. Turn out onto surface lightly dusted with sweet rice flour. Divide dough into 2 portions. Roll out each portion to about 1/8 inch (3 mm) thickness and line two 9-inch (23 cm) pie plates, or press dough directly into pie plates.

**Filling:** Mix first 3 ingredients in small bowl. Spread half into each pie crust.

Combine next 5 ingredients in a medium bowl. Pour half into each pie crust. Bake in preheated oven for 15 minutes. Reduce heat to 350°F (175°C) and bake for another 30 to 35 minutes until knife inserted in centre comes out clean.

*1 serving: 1046 Calories; 75 g Total Fat (15 g Mono, 3 g Poly, 35 g Sat); 447 mg Cholesterol; 59 g Carbohydrate; 3 g Fibre; 34 g Protein; 1490 mg Sodium*

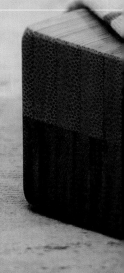

## Filling

**15 bacon slices, cooked crisp and crumbled**

**2 cups (500 mL) shredded Swiss cheese**

**2/3 cup (150 mL) finely chopped onion**

**8 large eggs, fork-beaten**

**4 cups (1 L) half-and-half cream**

**1 1/2 tsp (7 mL) salt**

**1/2 tsp (2 mL) sugar**

**1/4 tsp (1 mL) cayenne pepper**

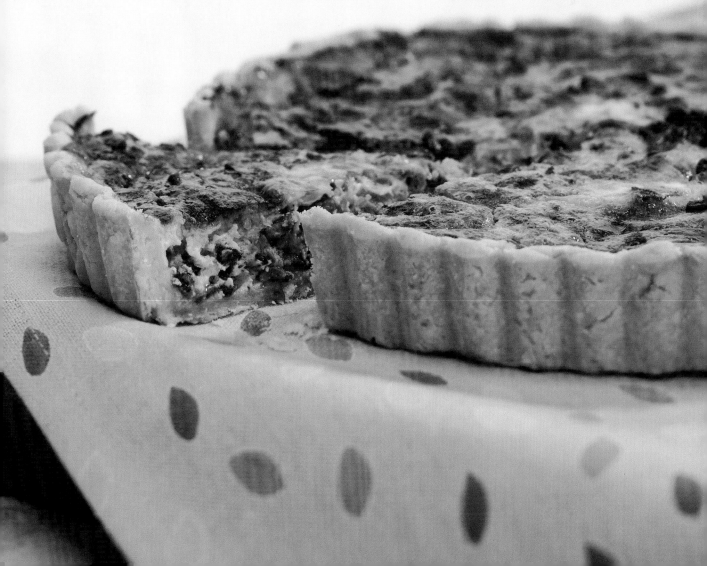

# Potato Leek Casserole

## Serves 8 to 12

In Germany, we had many dishes that combined leeks and potatoes, and this one is still a favourite. If you can't find leeks, try using sweet onions instead, although leeks are still the best in this casserole. Use smoked bacon for the right flavour.

**6 medium potatoes, cut into 1/2 inch (12 mm) cubes**

**5 to 6 sprigs of fresh thyme**

**5 garlic cloves**

**1 1/2 tsp (7 mL) salt**

**15 bacon slices**

**6 leeks (white part only), halved and cut into 1/2 inch (12 mm) pieces**

**3 Tbsp (45 mL) butter**

**1 1/2 tsp (7 mL) salt**

**1 tsp (5 mL) pepper**

**15 large eggs**

**4 cups (1 L) half-and-half cream**

**3 cups (750 mL) grated Swiss cheese**

**1 1/2 tsp (7 mL) ground nutmeg**

**3 cups (750 mL) grated Swiss cheese**

Preheat oven to 325°F (160°C). Grease a 9 x 13 inch (23 x 33 cm) baking pan. Place first 4 ingredients in a large pot. Add water until potatoes are just covered. Bring to a boil. Cook for 5 to 6 minutes until just starting to soften. Remove from heat. Drain. Discard garlic and thyme.

Cook bacon in a large frying pan until crisp. Transfer with slotted spoon to paper towel–lined plate to drain. Crumble bacon pieces and set aside. Drain and discard all but 1 1/2 Tbsp (25 mL) drippings. Add next 4 ingredients. Cook on medium for 9 to 12 minutes until leeks are softened. Add potatoes and stir.

Beat eggs in a large bowl until frothy. Slowly add cream, potato mixture, bacon, first amount of cheese and nutmeg. Spread evenly into prepared pan. Cover with foil and bake in preheated oven for 50 to 60 minutes until set and knife inserted in centre comes out clean.

Sprinkle second amount of cheese over casserole. Broil, uncovered, for 2 to 4 minutes until cheese is browned. Let stand for 8 to 12 minutes before serving.

*1 serving*: 855 Calories; 54 g Total Fat (17 g Mono, 3 g Poly, 30 g Sat); 405 mg Cholesterol; 49 g Carbohydrate; 5 g Fibre; 44 g Protein; 1375 mg Sodium

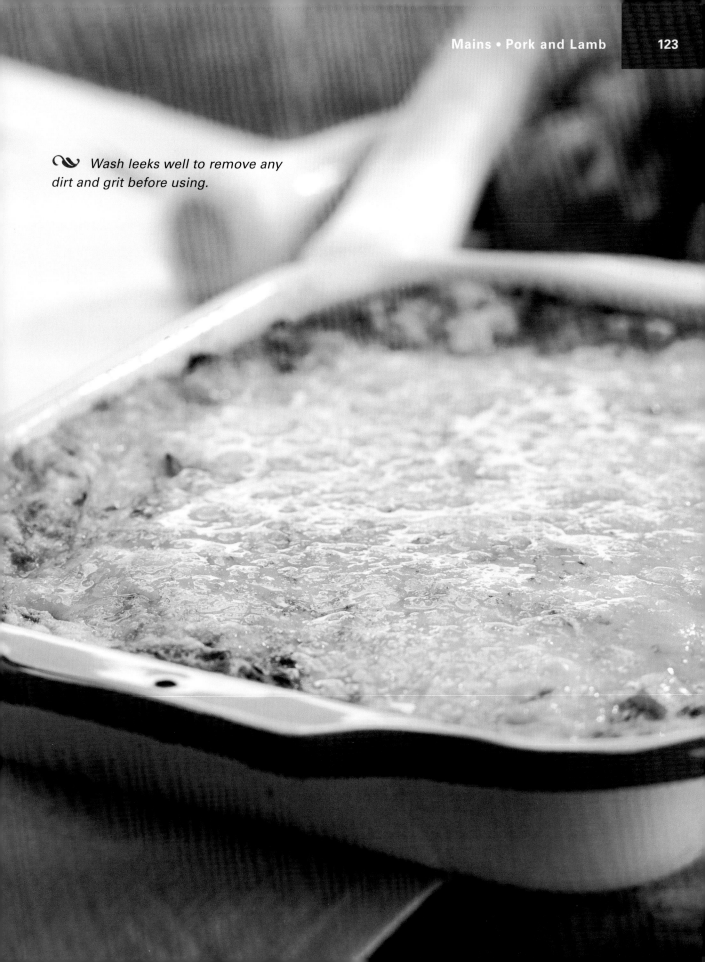

*Wash leeks well to remove any dirt and grit before using.*

# Lemon Pork Wrap

## Serves 6

Wrap some flavourful pork in a soft tortilla, top with salad dressing and add some cheese, and you have a handy meal when you're on the go.

## Wraps

1/3 cup (75 mL) pea starch

1/3 cup (75 mL) sweet rice flour

1/3 cup (75 mL) tapioca starch

2 Tbsp (30 mL) whey powder

1 1/2 Tbsp (25 mL) pea fibre III

2 1/2 tsp (12 mL) baking powder

2 tsp (10 mL) xanthan gum

1 1/4 tsp (6 mL) guar gum

1/4 tsp (1 mL) salt

2 cups (500 mL) milk

4 large eggs, room temperature

1 egg white (large)

2 Tbsp (30 mL) cooking oil

2 tsp (10 mL) cooking oil, *divided*

(continued on next page)

**Wraps:** Mix first 9 ingredients in a medium metal bowl.

Mix next 4 ingredients in a separate bowl. Combine wet ingredients with dry ingredients and knead together or use a heavy-duty mixer with a dough hook attachment.

Preheat griddle to medium-high (if you don't own a griddle, use a very flat, unwarped frying pan and heat on stovetop). Heat 1 tsp (5 mL) cooking oil on griddle until hot. Pour batter onto griddle, using about 1/3 cup (75 mL) for each wrap. Cook for 1 to 2 minutes until bubbles form on top. Turn wrap over. Cook for 1 to 2 minutes until brown. Repeat with remaining batter, heating more cooking oil on griddle with each batch if necessary to prevent sticking.

**Filling:** Heat cooking oil in a frying pan on medium-high. Add pork. Cook until all sides are browned. Add remaining 5 ingredients. Cook for 15 to 20 minutes, stirring occasionally, until desired doneness.

Place filling, lettuce, salad dressing and cheese on each wrap. Fold wrap.

*1 serving (without toppings): 394 Calories; 18 g Total Fat (9 g Mono, 3 g Poly, 4 g Sat); 195 mg Cholesterol; 28 g Carbohydrate; 3 g Fibre; 30 g Protein; 841 mg Sodium*

(continued on next page)

**Honey Mustard Chicken Wraps:** Omit pork. Replace with 6 x 4 to 6 oz (113 to 170 g) boneless, skinless chicken breast halves, cut into 1/4-inch (6 mm) cubes. Omit maple syrup, lemon juice, lemon pepper and marjoram. Replace with 2 Tbsp (30 mL) honey, 1 Tbsp (15 mL) Dijon mustard, 1 Tbsp (15 mL) Italian seasoning, 2 tsp (10 mL) poultry seasoning and 1 tsp (5 mL) pepper.

## Filling

1 Tbsp (15 mL) cooking oil

6 x 4 to 6 oz (113 to 170 g) medium boneless pork fillets, cut into small cubes

1 Tbsp (15 mL) maple syrup

juice from 1 large lemon

1 tsp (5 mL) lemon pepper

1 tsp (5 mL) dried marjoram

1 tsp (5 mL) salt

cut or torn romaine lettuce, lightly packed

Ranch (or Caesar) salad dressing

grated medium Cheddar cheese

# Rosemary Lamb Chops

## Serves 6

Fresh rosemary and the oil-vinegar marinade offer a typical time-tested Mediterranean taste profile to these tender lamb chops. These present well with rice, Brussels sprouts and garlic bread sticks and will offer a meat alternative to your staple meat fare of beef, chicken and pork.

**1/2 cup (125 mL) balsamic vinegar**

**6 Tbsp (90 mL) olive oil**

**6 garlic cloves, minced**

**1/4 cup (60 mL) dry red wine**

**3 Tbsp (45 mL) lemon juice**

**3 Tbsp (45 mL) fresh rosemary, or 1 Tbsp (15 mL) dried, crushed**

**1 Tbsp (15 mL) gluten-free teriyaki sauce (see page 156)**

**1 tsp (5 mL) pepper**

**12 lamb loin chops, about 1 inch (2.5 cm) thick, trimmed of fat**

Combine first 8 ingredients.

Place lamb chops in a large bowl or dish with a tightly fitting lid. Pour vinegar mixture over top. Chill, covered, for 5 hours or overnight. Flip container occasionally to coat chops completely. Drain and discard marinade. Cook lamb chops on greased grill for about 5 minutes per side until desired doneness.

*1 serving: 338 Calories; 21 g Total Fat (13 g Mono, 2 g Poly, 5 g Sat); 86 mg Cholesterol; 5 g Carbohydrate; 0 g Fibre; 28 g Protein; 129 mg Sodium*

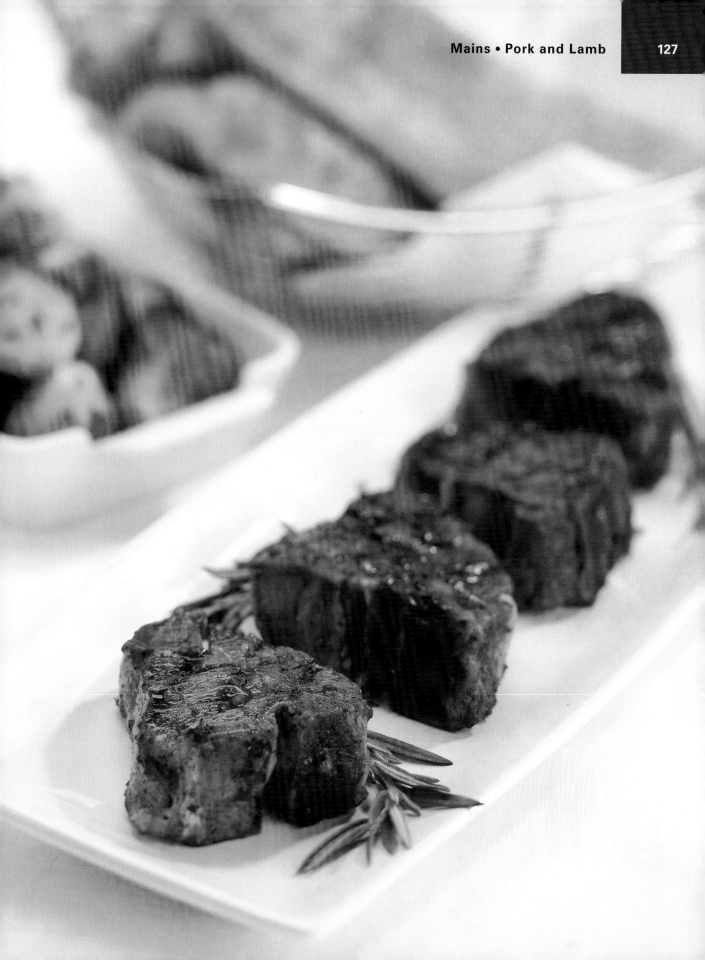

# Quinoa Casserole

## Serves 6 to 8

Quinoa, the powerful, nutritious gluten-free grain, forms the base for this cheese and vegetable casserole for a satisfying vegetarian dish that's packed with protein.

**1 1/2 cups (375 mL) quinoa, rinsed and drained**

**3 cups (750 mL) water or vegetable stock**

**1 cup (250 mL) broccoli florets**

**8 large eggs, fork-beaten**

**1 cup (250 mL) finely chopped spinach**

**1 cup (250 mL) grated medium Cheddar cheese**

**1/3 cup (75 mL) half-and-half cream**

**1 to 2 tsp (5 to 10 mL) garlic and herb no-salt seasoning (such as Mrs. Dash)**

Preheat oven to 350°F (175°C). Combine quinoa and water in a small pot on medium-high. Bring to a boil. Cook, uncovered, for about 15 minutes until tender. Spread evenly into a lightly greased 9 x 13 inch (23 x 33 cm) or 10 inch (25 cm) square baking pan.

Process broccoli in food processor until finely ground but not mushy. Combine broccoli and next 5 ingredients in a medium bowl. Spread over quinoa. Bake in preheated oven for 25 to 35 minutes until golden brown.

*1 serving:* 325 Calories; 16 g Total Fat (5 g Mono, 1 g Poly, 7 g Sat); 307 mg Cholesterol; 26 g Carbohydrate; 3 g Fibre; 19 g Protein; 346 mg Sodium

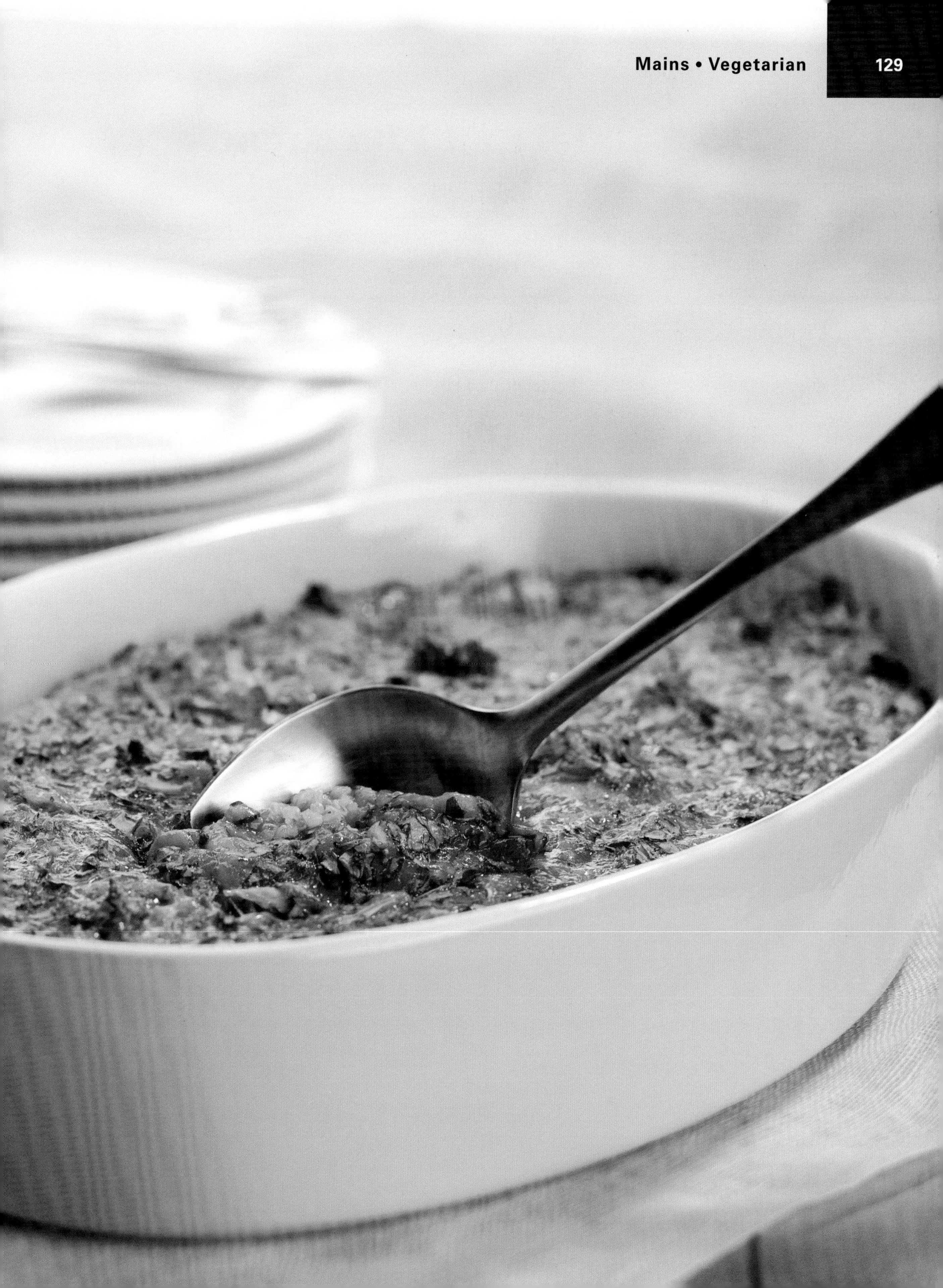

# Falafel and Pita Bread

## Serves 6 to 8

A Mediterranean staple and a favourite of mine. Make sure to chop the onion very finely. Enjoy in a gluten-free pita wrap along with veggies, hummus or tahini sauce, yogurt and rice. The bread is best eaten fresh and doesn't store for long.

**1/4 to 1/2 cup (60 to 125 mL) canola or sunflower oil**

## Falafel

**1 x 14 oz (398 mL) can chickpeas, drained**

**1 medium onion, finely chopped**

**2 to 3 Tbsp (30 to 45 mL) gluten-free all-purpose flour (see page 9)**

**2 Tbsp (30 mL) finely chopped fresh parsley**

**1 Tbsp (15 mL) crushed garlic**

**1 tsp (5 mL) ground coriander**

**3/4 tsp (4 mL) ground cumin**

**1/2 tsp (2 mL) salt**

*(continued on next page)*

Heat canola oil to 350°F (175°C) in a pot or deep fryer, according to manufacturer's instructions.

**Falafel:** Place next 8 ingredients in a food processor and grind into a thick paste. Roll mixutre into 1 1/2 to 2 inch (4 to 5 cm) balls. Flatten slightly. Deep-fry, in batches, in hot oil for 3 to 4 minutes per batch until cooked through. Transfer to paper towel–lined plate to drain. Cover to keep warm.

*(continued on next page)*

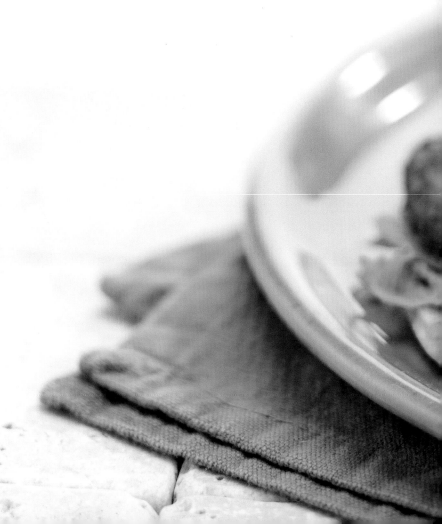

**Pita Bread:** Mix first 11 ingredients in a medium metal bowl.

Mix remaining 4 ingredients in a separate bowl. Add egg mixture to flour mixture. Knead together or use a heavy-duty mixer with a dough hook attachment. Turn out dough onto surface lightly dusted with sweet rice flour. Divide dough into 2 balls. Roll dough pieces out very thinly. Cut into 8 to 10 inch (20 to 25 cm) rounds. Cook in ungreased cast-iron pan or nonstick griddle on medium and heat on each side. The dough will separate in the middle and an air bubble will appear, creating a "pocket." Serve falafel wrapped in pita bread.

*1 serving: 393 Calories; 18 g Total Fat (10 g Mono, 4 g Poly, 2 g Sat); 38 mg Cholesterol; 52 g Carbohydrate; 7 g Fibre; 9 g Protein; 602 mg Sodium*

## Pita Bread

2/3 cup (150 mL) sweet rice flour

2/3 cup (150 mL) tapioca starch

1/3 cup (75 mL) pea starch

2 Tbsp (30 mL) sugar

2 Tbsp (30 mL) whey powder

1 1/2 Tbsp (25 mL) active dry yeast

1 1/2 Tbsp (25 mL) pea fibre III

2 tsp (10 mL) baking powder

2 tsp (10 mL) xanthan gum

1 1/4 tsp (6 mL) guar gum

1/4 tsp (1 mL) salt

1/2 cup (125 mL) water

3 Tbsp (45 mL) cooking oil

2 egg whites (large), room temperature

1 large egg, room temperature

# Crustless Broccoli Quiche

## Serves 6

This crustless quiche provides a pleasant all-in-one meal with the complementary combination of broccoli, cheese and subtle herbs. You can also divide the filling into smaller pans for individual servings—just decrease baking time a bit in this case.

6 large eggs, fork-beaten

1 cup (250 mL) grated medium Cheddar cheese

1 cup (250 mL) finely chopped broccoli florets

1/2 cup (125 mL) half-and-half cream

1/3 cup (75 mL) brown rice flour

1 to 2 tsp (5 to 10 mL) salt

1/4 tsp (1 mL) dried marjoram

1/4 tsp (1 mL) dried oregano

1/4 tsp (1 mL) dried thyme

1/8 tsp (0.5 mL) pepper

Preheat oven to 350°F (175°C). Place all 10 ingredients in a large bowl and mix well. Spread mixture evenly in a greased 9-inch (23 cm) deep pie plate. Bake in oven for 35 to 40 minutes until set and knife inserted in centre comes out clean.

*1 serving: 213 Calories; 14 g Total Fat (4 g Mono, 1 g Poly, 7 g Sat); 239 mg Cholesterol; 9 g Carbohydrate; 0 g Fibre; 13 g Protein; 588 mg Sodium*

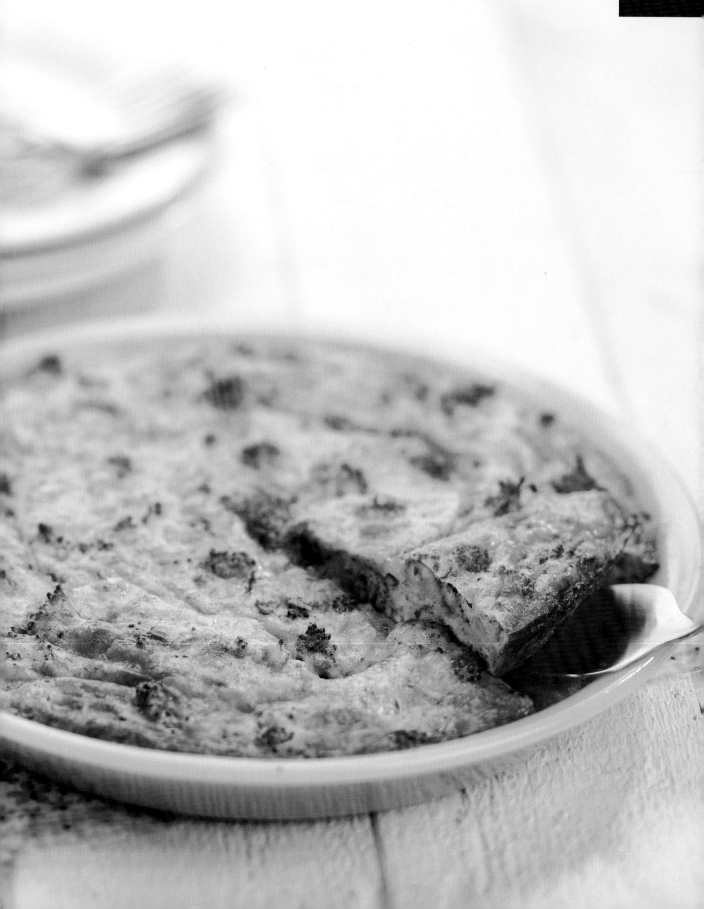

# Walnut Lentil Burgers

## Makes 6 to 8

1 1/2 cups (375 mL) brown lentils

1 1/2 cups (375 mL) whole walnuts, toasted

2 large eggs, fork-beaten, room temperature

1 small onion, finely chopped

1/2 cup (125 mL) gluten-free bread crumbs (see page 9)

1/3 cup (75 mL) finely grated carrot

2 Tbsp (30 mL) brown rice flour

1 tsp (5 mL) dried rosemary, crushed

1 tsp (5 mL) gluten-free soy sauce

1 tsp (5 mL) salt

1/2 tsp (2 mL) pepper

1/3 to 1/2 cup (75 to 125 mL) cooking oil

6 to 8 gluten-free hamburger buns

Prepare lentils according to package directions. Let cool. Process lentils and walnuts in food processor until finely chopped but not mushy. Transfer to a large bowl.

Add next 9 ingredients. Mix well. Shape into patties 3 inches (7.5 cm) wide and 1/2 inch (12 mm) thick.

Heat cooking oil in a frying pan on medium. Add patties to frying pan. Cook for 3 to 5 minutes per side until cooked through. Serve patties in buns with your favourite toppings, like lettuce, tomato or pineapple.

*1 serving (with bun):* 703 Calories; 42 g Total Fat (11 g Mono, 17 g Poly, 4 g Sat); 71 mg Cholesterol; 64 g Carbohydrate; 11 g Fibre; 22 g Protein; 663 mg Sodium

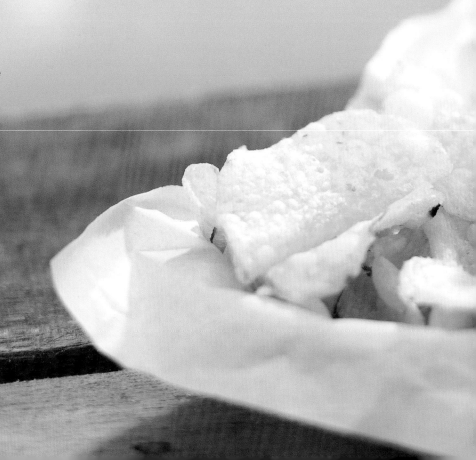

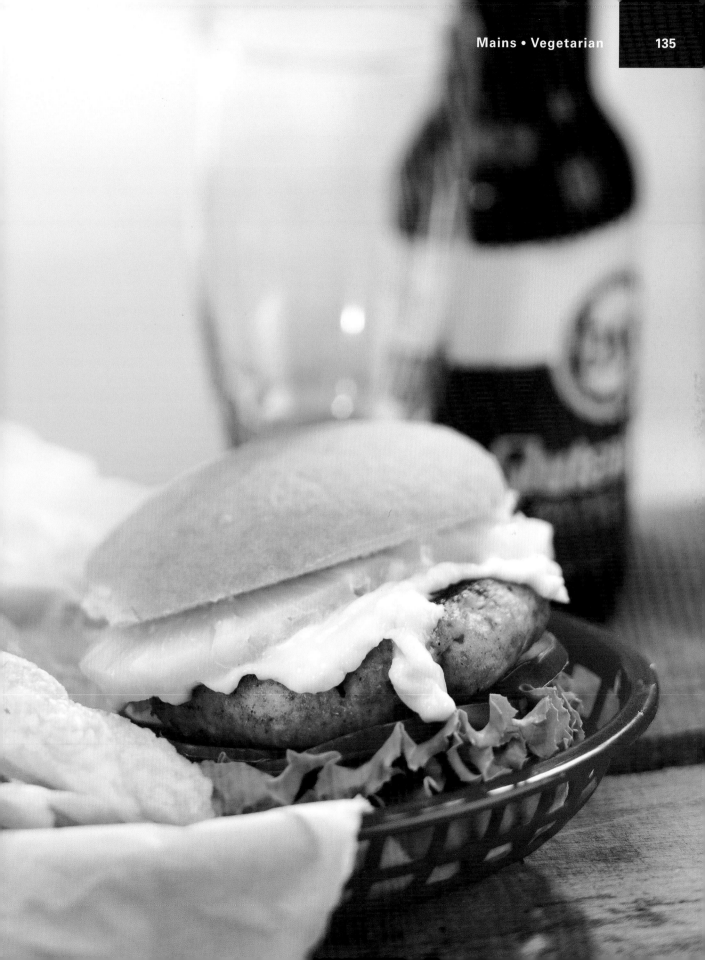

# Veggie Calzones

## Makes 1 large, 2 medium or 6 small

A traditional large pizza pocket filled with your favourites—basically kind of like a folded-over pizza. You can make the calzones large or divide the dough into several portions to make smaller ones. or you can roll the dough out and make a layer pizza. (see cover photo).

## Dough

2/3 cup (150 mL) sweet rice flour

2/3 cup (150 mL) tapioca starch

1/3 cup (75 mL) pea starch

2 Tbsp (30 mL) sugar

2 Tbsp (30 mL) whey powder

1 1/2 Tbsp (25 mL) active dry yeast

1 1/2 Tbsp (25 mL) pea fibre III

2 tsp (10 mL) xanthan gum

1 1/4 tsp (6 mL) guar gum

1/4 tsp (1 mL) salt

1/2 cup (125 mL) water

3 Tbsp (45 mL) cooking oil

1 large egg, room temperature

1 egg white (large)

(continued on next page)

**Dough:** Preheat oven to 350°F (175°C). Mix first 10 ingredients in a medium metal bowl.

Mix next 4 ingredients in a separate bowl. Add egg mixture to flour mixture. Knead together or use a heavy-duty mixer with a dough hook attachment. Turn out dough onto surface lightly dusted with sweet rice flour. Divide dough into 2 or more balls, depending on the desired size of calzones. Roll dough pieces out to an appropriate thickness.

**Filling:** Heat oil in a large frying pan on medium. Add broccoli. Cook for 1 to 2 minutes until broccoli is tender-crisp. Remove from heat. Add next 6 ingredients. Stir. Add filling evenly to the centre of dough pieces. Fold dough over and pinch edges to seal.

**Egg Wash:** Combine egg and milk or water in a small bowl. Brush calzones with egg wash. Place calzones on greased baking sheet in preheated oven for 30 to 35 minutes or until desired browning. If making a flat pizza, bake for 20-25 minutes or until desired browning.

*1 small calzone: 430 Calories; 23 g Total Fat (10 g Mono, 4 g Poly, 7 g Sat); 103 mg Cholesterol; 42 g Carbohydrate; 5 g Fibre; 18 g Protein; 457 mg Sodium*

(continued on next page)

**Pepperoni Calzones:** For filling, combine 3/4 cup (175 mL) gluten-free pizza sauce, 1/2 cup (125 mL) cubed pepperoni and 1 1/4 cups (300 mL) grated mozzarella cheese.

**Hawaiian Calzones:** For filling, combine 3/4 cup (175 mL) gluten-free pizza sauce, 1/2 cup (125 mL) cubed deli ham, 1/3 cup (75 mL) pineapple pieces and 1 1/4 cups (300 mL) grated mozzarella cheese.

**BBQ Chicken Calzones:** For filling, combine 3/4 cup (175 mL) gluten-free barbecue sauce, 3/4 cup (175 mL) cubed cooked chicken, 4 to 6 bacon slices (cooked crisp and crumbled) and 1 1/2 cups (375 mL) mozzarella cheese.

## Filling

2 to 3 Tbsp (30 to 45 mL) cooking oil

1 1/2 cups (375 mL) chopped broccoli florets

3/4 cup (175 mL) grated mozzarella cheese

1/2 cup (125 mL) grated provolone cheese

1/2 cup (125 mL) ricotta cheese

1/4 cup (60 mL) grated Parmesan cheese

1/2 tsp (2 mL) Italian seasoning

1/2 tsp (2 mL) garlic powder

## Egg Wash

1 large egg, fork-beaten

1/2 cup (125 mL) milk or water

# Chickpea Masala with Garlic Bread

## Serves 6 to 8

An Asian-influenced vegetarian dish served with a side of garlic bread—I find this an excellent taste combination. For convenience, this recipe uses canned chickpeas. Sometimes I substitute smaller chana dal (hulled lentils or beans) for the more traditional chickpeas. You can make garlic bread easily by starting with store-bought gluten-free bread, or you can make it from scratch with the recipe below.

## Garlic Bread

1/4 cup (60 mL) warm water

1 Tbsp (15 mL) active dry yeast

2 tsp (10 mL) sugar


1 1/2 cups (375 mL) tapioca starch

1 1/2 cups (375 mL) white rice flour

1/4 cup (60 mL) whey powder

2 Tbsp (30 mL) pea fibre 80

2 Tbsp (30 mL) sugar

4 tsp (20 mL) xanthan gum

1 tsp (5 mL) dough improver (see page 9)

1 tsp (15 mL) salt


1 3/4 cups (425 mL) water

1/2 cup (125 mL) egg whites (from 4 large eggs), room temperature


1/2 cup (125 mL) butter, softened

2 garlic cloves, minced

1 1/2 tsp (7 mL) chopped fresh parsley

*(continued on next page)*

**Garlic Bread:** Place first 3 ingredients in a small bowl.

Mix next 8 ingredients in a large bowl.

Mix water and egg whites in a separate bowl. Add egg white mixture and yeast mixture to flour mixture. Mix until a smooth batter is formed. Pour batter into a greased 9 x 5 inch (23 x 12.5 cm) baking pan and smooth with a wet spatula. Place in a warm place and cover with a damp towel. Let rise until doubled in size. Place pans in a 350°F (175°C) oven on middle rack. Bake for 50 minutes until bread sounds hollow when tapped on bottom. Remove from oven and place on a wire rack to cool.

Combine butter, garlic and parsley in a small bowl. Cut bread into slices and spread with garlic butter. Place bread slices on a baking pan. Bake in preheated oven for 10 to 15 minutes until golden brown.

*(continued on next page)*

**Masala:** Heat oil in a large saucepan on medium. Add onion. Cook for about 5 minutes, stirring often, until onion is softened. Add garlic and ginger. Cook for about 2 minutes until fragrant.

Add next 5 ingredients. Stir well. Simmer for 2 minutes.

Slowly add next 4 ingredients, stirring constantly. Cook for 15 to 20 minutes, stirring occasionally, until mixture is thickened.

Add lime and vinegar and stir. Serve with garlic bread.

*1 serving (with bread): 871 Calories; 34 g Total Fat (9 g Mono, 3 g Poly, 18 g Sat); 46 mg Cholesterol; 122 g Carbohydrate; 19 g Fibre; 24 g Protein; 1133 mg Sodium*

## Masala

3 Tbsp (45 mL) canola oil

2 medium onions, finely diced

6 garlic cloves, minced

2 Tbsp (30 mL) grated ginger root

2 tsp (10 mL) curry powder

2 tsp (10 mL) ground coriander

2 tsp (10 mL) ground cumin

2 tsp (10 mL) garam masala

1/4 tsp (1 mL) salt

1 cup (250 mL) coconut milk

1/2 to 3/4 cup (125 to 175 mL) tomato paste

2 tsp (10 mL) dark buckwheat honey

2 x 19 oz (540 mL) cans of chickpeas (garbanzo beans), rinsed and drained

1 Tbsp (15 mL) lime juice

1 Tbsp (15 mL) rice vinegar

# Mac 'n' Cheese

## Serves 6

Everyone loves comfort food. Kids (and adults) of all ages love this version of macaroni and cheese. In my family, sometimes we skip the baking step and just eat the pasta and sauce straight from the stove, adding in some steamed broccoli. The baked version of the recipe is especially good on cool or cloudy days.

**4 cups (1 L) gluten-free corn elbow macaroni**

Preheat oven to 350°F (175°C). Grease a 9 x 13 inch (23 x 33 cm) baking pan. Cook pasta according to package directions to *al dente.* Drain. Return to same pot. Cover to keep warm.

**6 Tbsp (90 mL) butter**

**1/4 cup (60 mL) gluten-free all-purpose flour (see page 9)**

**1 tsp (5 mL) salt**

**1/8 tsp (0.5 mL) pepper**

Melt butter in a medium saucepan on medium. Add flour, salt and pepper. Cook for 1 minute, stirring often.

**2 cups (500 mL) milk**

**2 cups (500 mL) half-and-half cream**

**4 to 5 cups (1 to 1.25 L) cubed medium Cheddar cheese**

Slowly add milk and cream, stirring constantly. Cook for 3 to 5 minutes until thickened. Add cheese a bit at a time, stirring until melted before adding more. Add cheese mixture to pasta. Stir until coated. Transfer to prepared baking pan. Bake in preheated oven for 30 to 40 minutes until top is slightly crispy.

*1 serving:* 845 Calories; 47 g Total Fat (13 g Mono, 2 g Poly, 29 g Sat); 143 mg Cholesterol; 74 g Carbohydrate; 1 g Fibre; 31 g Protein; 1045 mg Sodium

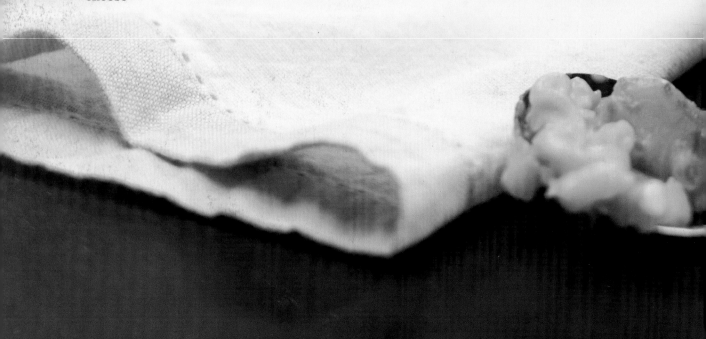

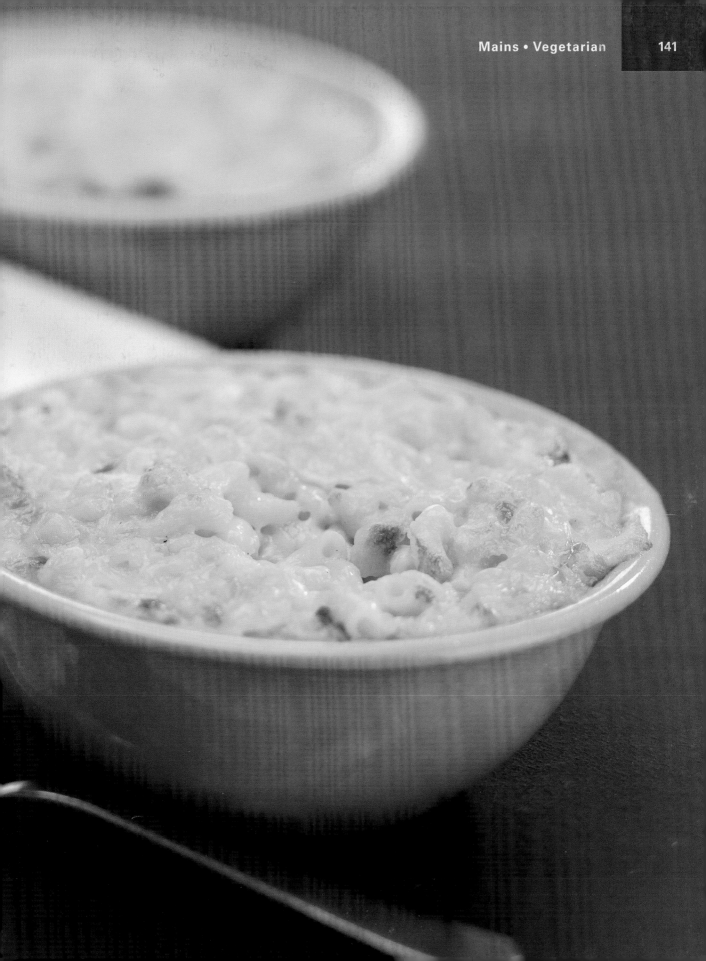

# Spaetzle

## Serves 6

This famous noodle dish is great with savoury meat entrées like Wiener Schnitzel (see page 112) and is often accompanied by red cabbage and gravy. Spaetzle can be used as a pasta substitute in many dishes. This recipe uses a spaetzle board by the Nana company (www.cookingwithnana.com), which was developed specifically for spaetzle (see Tip, page 143).

**1 cup (250 mL) sweet rice flour**

**3/4 cup (175 mL) pea starch**

**1/2 cup (125 mL) brown rice flour**

**1/2 cup (125 mL) white rice flour**

**4 large eggs, room temperature**

**1/2 cup (125 mL) water, approximately**

**16 cups (4 L) water**

Combine first 5 ingredients in a medium bowl. Mix well. Slowly add first amount of water to form a soft dough.

Bring second amount of water to a boil in a large saucepan or Dutch oven. Reduce heat to medium. Place spaetzle board on top of pot. Scrape small balls of dough back and forth over the board. Cook for 3 to 4 minutes until noodles float to the top. Drain. You can plunge the noodles into ice water to cool them off if desired. I simply add a bit of butter to prevent them from sticking together. Spaeztle can be further cooked in a frying pan for 5 to 6 minutes until golden brown, adding herbs and spices to taste.

*1 serving*: 286 Calories; 4 g Total Fat (1 g Mono, 1 g Poly, 1 g Sat); 141 mg Cholesterol; 49 g Carbohydrate; 7 g Fibre; 13 g Protein; 51 mg Sodium

## Tip

A spaetzle board is specially designed to drip dough in small globules into boiling water. It looks like a plastic frying pan, but with a wavy bottom and small holes throughout. It usually comes with a "scraper" to help push the dough through the holes. If you don't have a spaetzle board, you can use a box cheese grater and a spatula to achieve the same result (though with a bit more mess).

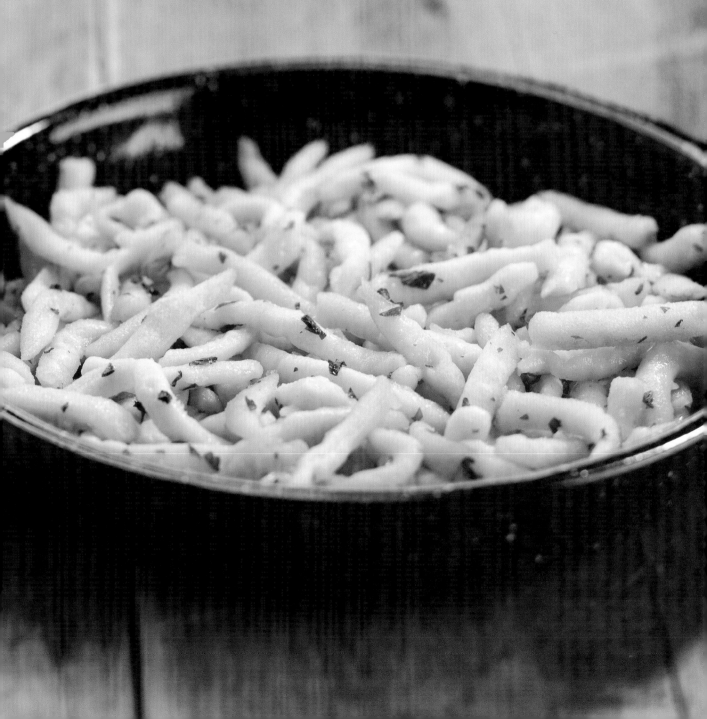

# Pilaf

## Serves 6

Pilaf can be served as a side or as a main dish. Traditionally made with rice and a variety of vegetable or meat additions, spices and herbs, pilaf is a staple in many countries.

**1/4 cup (60 mL) chopped green onions**

**2 garlic cloves, minced**

**1/4 cup (60 mL) butter or margarine, softened**

**1 1/2 cups (375 mL) long-grain rice**

**1/4 tsp (1 mL) garam masala**

**3 cups (750 mL) chicken broth**

**1/2 tsp (2 mL) salt**

**1/2 cup (125 mL) Thompson raisins**

**1/2 cup (125 mL) chopped almonds, toasted**

**1/4 cup (60 mL) chopped green onions**

Cook first amount of green onions and garlic in butter in a large skillet on medium for 3 to 5 minutes, stirring occasionally, until tender. Add rice and garam masala. Cook for 2 to 3 minutes, stirring constantly, until rice is lightly browned.

Heat chicken broth and salt in a saucepan on medium for 5 to 7 minutes until hot. Pour over rice mixture. Stir. Simmer, covered, on low for 35 to 40 minutes until rice is tender. Remove from heat.

Stir in raisins, almonds and second amount of green onions.

*1 serving: 344 Calories; 13 g Total Fat (5 g Mono, 2 g Poly, 5 g Sat); 20 mg Cholesterol; 52 g Carbohydrate; 2 g Fibre; 6 g Protein; 537 mg Sodium*

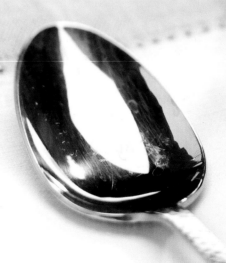

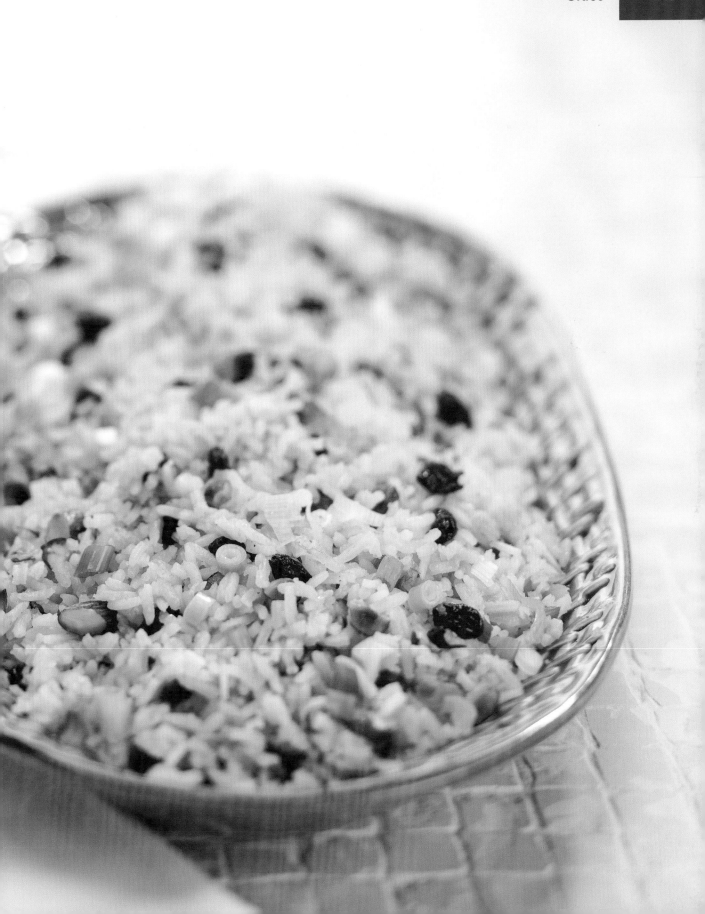

# Donna's Turnips and Apples

## Serves 8 to 12

I had never tasted this wonderful side dish until the fall of 2011. I know, you're telling me! Donna adjusted her recipe to make it gluten-free for me, and after several hours of tough negotiations, she agreed to let me add the recipe to this book. Like many great cooks, she does not really need precise measurements—a little bit of this, a little bit of that—so the following amounts for each ingredient are my translation of her suggestions. Prepare the yellow turnip and apple mixture at least a few hours or a day ahead of time, as it needs to cool.

**2 large yellow turnips (rutabagas), peeled and diced**

**1 tsp (5 mL) salt**

**2 Tbsp (30 mL) butter**

**1/4 cup (60 mL) half-and-half cream (or milk)**

**1/2 cup (125 mL) brown sugar**

**1/4 to 1/2 tsp (1 to 2 mL) ground cinnamon**

**3 large, firm apples (any varietal), peeled, cored and thinly sliced**

## Topping

**1/2 cup (125 mL) brown sugar**

**1/3 cup (75 mL) sweet rice flour**

**1/4 cup (60 mL) butter, softened**

Grease a 9 x 13 inch (23 x 33 cm) baking dish. Place yellow turnips in a pot. Add cold water to cover. Add salt. Cook on medium-high for 30 to 45 minutes until turnips are tender. Drain. Return turnips to pot. Add butter and cream. Mash. Add brown sugar and cinnamon.

Assemble in prepared baking dish as follows:

• 1/3 yellow turnip mixture

• 1/2 apple slices

• 1/3 yellow turnip mixture

• 1/2 apple slices

• 1/3 yellow turnip mixture

Chill, covered, for a few hours or overnight.

**Topping:** Preheat oven to 350°F (175°C). Mix remaining 3 ingredients until crumbs form. Sprinkle on top of yellow turnip and apple mixture. Bake in oven for 1 hour until top is golden brown and crisp. Serve hot.

*1 serving:* 244 Calories; 10 g Total Fat (2 g Mono, 0 g Poly, 6 g Sat); 26 mg Cholesterol; 40 g Carbohydrate; 2 g Fibre; 1 g Protein; 398 mg Sodium

*Yellow turnips are fairly firm and a bit harder to cut than potatoes. Using a large knife, first cut them in half, then into quarters, and then into small dice.*

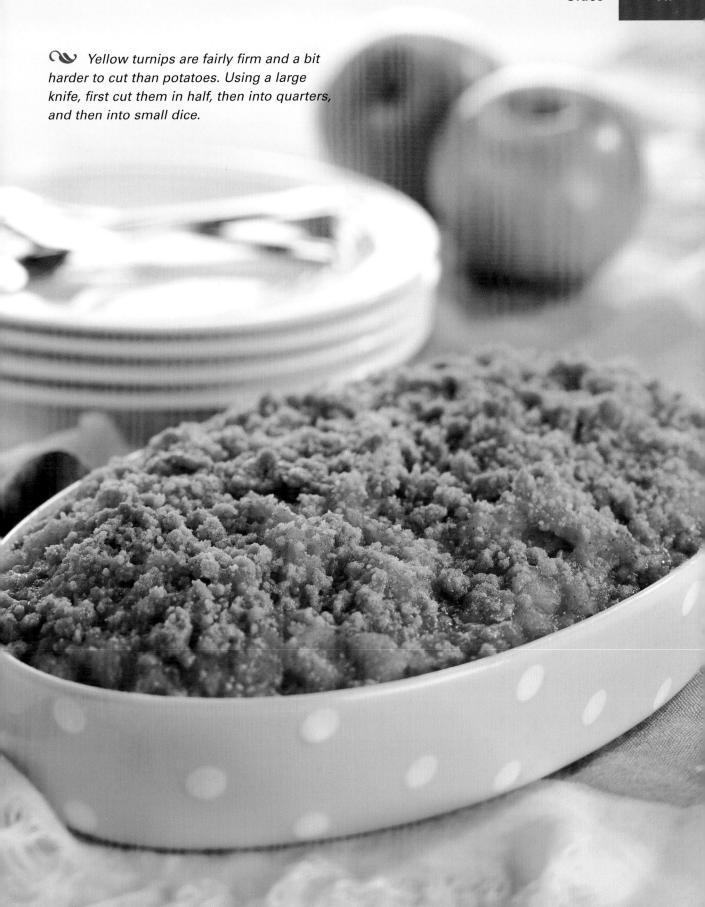

# Poultry Stuffing

## Serves 6 to 8

One of the best parts of any festive turkey, chicken or goose meal is the perfect stuffing. Legions of home cooks pride themselves on their stuffing, passed down from generation to generation. This stuffing combines the savoury notes of herbed bread cubes with the subtle flavours of orange, almonds and dried fruits. This recipe is the perfect amount for a 6 lb (2.7 kg) bird—adjust accordingly for the weight of your bird. You can substitute store-bought gluten-free herb bread, or use the recipe given here.

### Herb Bread

1/4 cup (60 mL) warm water

1 Tbsp (15 mL) active dry yeast

2 tsp (10 mL) sugar

1 1/2 cups (375 mL) cornstarch

1 1/2 cups (375 mL) white rice flour

1 Tbsp (15 mL) sugar

1 Tbsp (15 mL) xanthan gum

1 1/2 tsp (7 mL) baking powder

1 tsp (5 mL) dough improver (see page 9)

3/4 tsp (4 mL) salt

1 cup (250 mL) water

1/4 cup (60 mL) cooking oil

2 Tbsp (30 mL) honey

1 tsp (5 mL) dried oregano

1 tsp (5 mL) dried thyme

1/4 tsp (1 mL) black pepper

1/4 tsp (1 mL) Hungarian paprika

*(continued on next page)*

**Herb Bread:** Place first 3 ingredients in a small bowl. Let stand for 10 minutes until foamy.

Mix next 7 ingredients in a large bowl.

Mix next 3 ingredients in a separate bowl. Add honey mixture and yeast mixture to flour mixture.

Fold in remaining 4 ingredients. The dough will look like thick cake batter. Pour batter into a greased 9 x 5 inch (23 x 12.5 cm) baking pan. Smooth with a wet spatula. Place in a warm place and cover with a damp towel. Let rise for 15 to 25 minutes until about doubled in size. Bake on middle rack of a 350°F (175°C) oven for 50 to 60 until bread sounds hollow when tapped. Remove from oven and place on a wire rack to cool completely. Cut into thick slices. Cut into 3/4 inch (2 cm) cubes.

*(continued on next page)*

**Stuffing:** Combine bread cubes and remaining 9 ingredients. Fill bird cavity. Tie legs together with cooking twine. Cook bird as per instructions. Temperature of stuffing should reach at least 165°F (74°C).

*1 serving: 572 Calories; 18 g Total Fat (8 g Mono, 3 g Poly, 6 g Sat); 20 mg Cholesterol; 95 g Carbohydrate; 6 g Fibre; 4 g Protein; 461 mg Sodium*

## Stuffing

2 large apples, cored and chopped

1 medium red onion, chopped

5 dried apricots, chopped

5 pitted prunes, chopped

1 cup (250 mL) sliced seedless grapes

1/4 cup (60 mL) butter, melted

1/4 cup (60 mL) sake or mirin

2 to 3 Tbsp (30 to 45 mL) orange juice

2 to 3 tsp (10 to 15 mL) finely grated orange zest

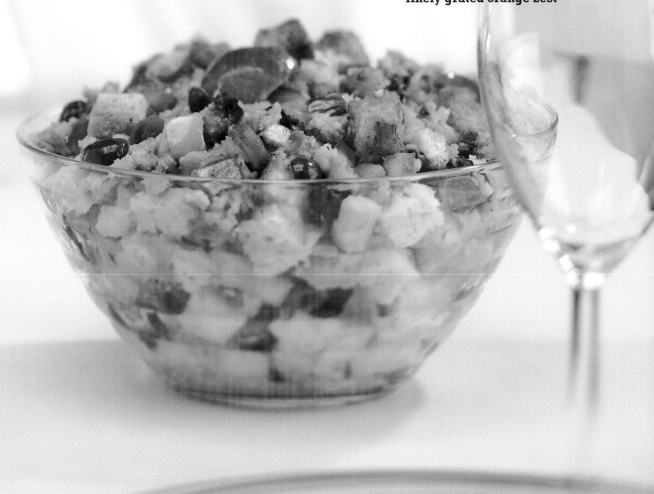

# Cornbread

## Serves 6 to 8

A traditional quickbread that can be a great side with meat or bean dishes. I also like to eat this cornbread fresh with Devonshire cream and Italian cherry jam.

**1 cup (250 mL) gluten-free all-purpose flour (see page 9)**

**1 cup (250 mL) fine cornmeal**

**1/3 cup (75 mL) sugar**

**1 Tbsp (15 mL) baking powder**

**3/4 tsp (4 mL) salt**

**1/3 cup (75 mL) canola oil**

**2 large eggs, room temperature**

**1 to 1 1/4 cups (250 to 300 mL) milk, room temperature**

Preheat oven to 400°F (200°C). Grease a 9 x 9 inch (23 x 23 cm) baking pan. Combine first 5 ingredients in a large bowl.

Combine remaining 3 ingredients in a medium bowl. Add milk mixture to flour mixture. Stir until just moistened. Pour batter into prepared pan. Bake in oven for 20 to 25 minutes until a knife inserted in centre of cornbread comes out clean.

*1 serving: 337 Calories; 15 g Total Fat (8 g Mono, 3 g Poly, 2 g Sat); 72 mg Cholesterol; 44 g Carbohydrate; 5 g Fibre; 7 g Protein; 495 mg Sodium*

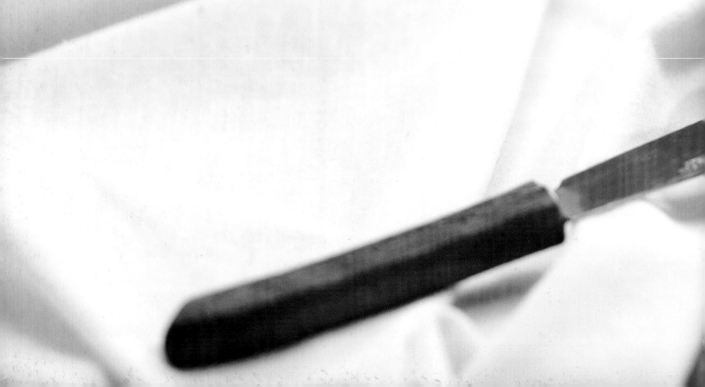

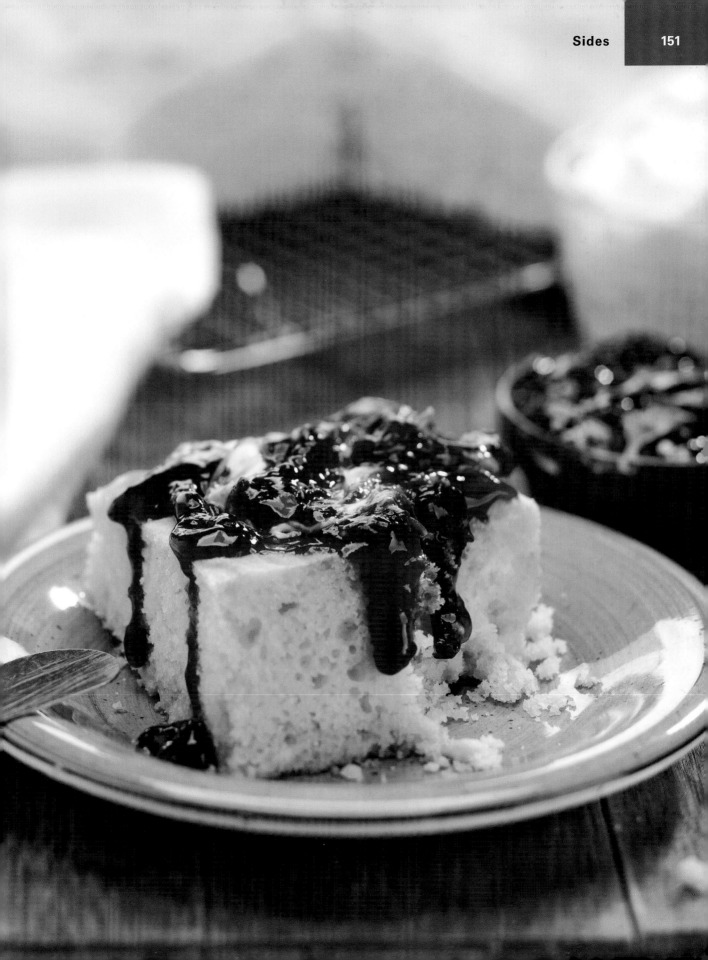

# Pommes de Terre au Gratin

## Serves 8 to 12

A very creamy, rich comfort food with layers of potatoes, cream, bacon and cheese. A perfect side dish to any festive dinner table or on any day all by itself.

**6 bacon slices, chopped**

**1 cup (250 mL) diced onions**

**6 large potatoes, about 3 lbs (1.4 kg), peeled, halved and thinly sliced**

**1 cup (250 mL) half-and-half cream**

**1 cup (250 mL) grated medium Cheddar cheese**

**1 cup (250 mL) grated mozzarella cheese**

**1 cup (250 mL) whipping cream**

**2 garlic cloves, minced**

**2 tsp (10 mL) salt**

**dash of cayenne pepper**

**1/3 cup (75 mL) grated Parmesan cheese**

Preheat oven to 400°F (200°C). Grease a 9 x 13 inch (23 x 33 cm) baking dish. Cook bacon in a large frying pan until golden. Add onion. Cook, stirring, until bacon is crispy. Remove from heat. Add potatoes. Mix well.

Combine next 7 ingredients in a large bowl. Layer ingredients in prepared dish as follows:

- 1/3 potato mixture
- 1/3 cream mixture
- 1/3 potato mixture
- 1/3 cream mixture
- 1/3 potato mixture
- 1/3 cream mixture

Top with Parmesan cheese. Baked in preheated oven for 40 to 45 minutes until potatoes are tender.

*1 serving*: 498 Calories; 25 g Total Fat (8 g Mono, 1 g Poly, 15 g Sat); 82 mg Cholesterol; 54 g Carbohydrate; 5 g Fibre; 18 g Protein; 925 mg Sodium

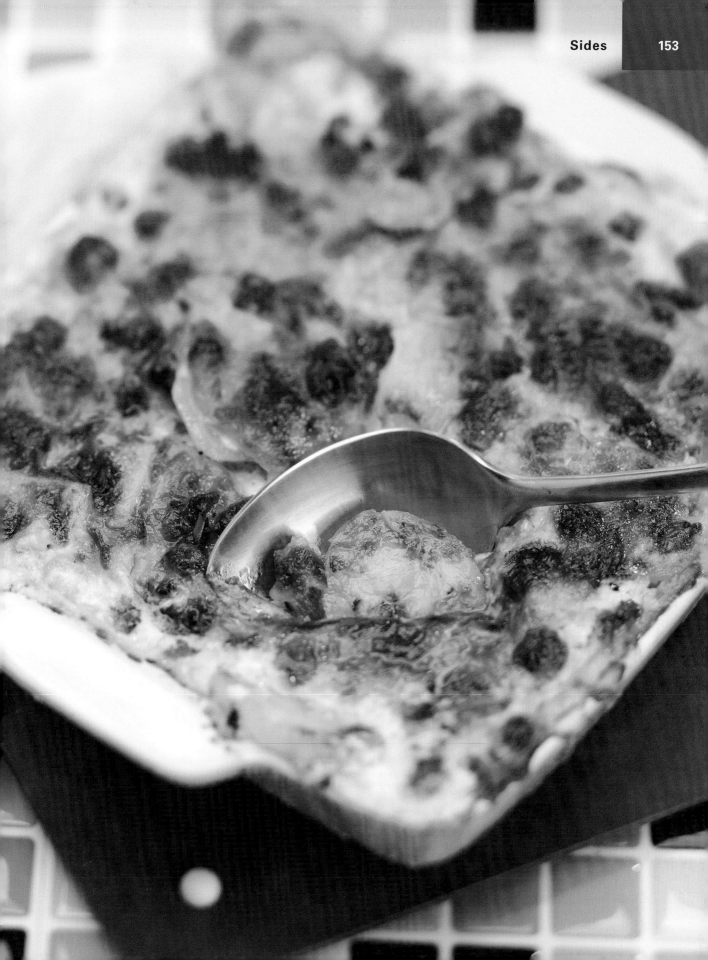

# Béchamel Sauce

## Makes about 6 cups

A classic sauce that elevates any meal. Can be used in pasta dishes, lasagna and many vegetable dishes. We used to have the sauce with boiled unpeeled whole potatoes (Pell Kartoffel) and quark (a soft cheese) as a main dish in Europe.

**4 cups (1 L) milk**

**1 medium onion, quartered**

**3 to 5 whole cloves**

**2 bay leaves**

Heat first 4 ingredients in a small saucepan on medium for 10 to 15 minutes. Remove and discard onion, bay leaves and cloves.

**1/2 cup (125 mL) butter**

**1/2 to 3/4 cup (125 to 175 mL) gluten-free all-purpose flour (see page 9)**

Melt butter in a saucepan on medium. Whisk in flour. Adjust amount of flour according to desired consistency. Heat and stir for 1 minute.

Slowly add milk to flour mixture, whisking constantly until thickened. Add salt, pepper and nutmeg. Stir.

*1 cup: 261 Calories; 17 g Total Fat (4 g Mono, 1 g Poly, 11 g Sat); 47 mg Cholesterol; 20 g Carbohydrate; 0 g Fibre; 8 g Protein; 317 mg Sodium*

**1/4 tsp (1 mL) salt**

**1/4 tsp (1 mL) pepper**

**1/8 tsp (0.5 mL) ground nutmeg**

# Brown Meat Gravy

## Makes about 3 cups

Using the drippings from your cooked roast, poultry or steak, you can make a nice gravy with this simple method. Adjust the amounts of flour and liquid until you reach the desired consistency.

**1/4 to 1/3 cup (60 to 75 mL) drippings**

**3 to 4 Tbsp (45 to 60 mL) gluten-free all-purpose flour (see page 9)**

**1 1/4 cup (300 mL) milk**

**1 1/4 cup (300 mL) water**

**1/2 to 1 tsp (2 to 5 mL) salt**

**1/8 to 1/4 tsp (0.5 to 1 mL) pepper**

Heat drippings in a small pot or roasting pan on medium. Add flour. Heat for about 1 minute, constantly stirring, until brown. Slowly add milk, stirring constantly. Scrape any brown bits from bottom of pan. Slowly add water. Cook, stirring constantly, until gravy is thickened. Add salt and pepper to taste.

*1 cup: 227 Calories; 18 g Total Fat (7 g Mono, 1 g Poly, 8 g Sat); 21 mg Cholesterol; 11 g Carbohydrate; 1 g Fibre; 5 g Protein; 549 mg Sodium*

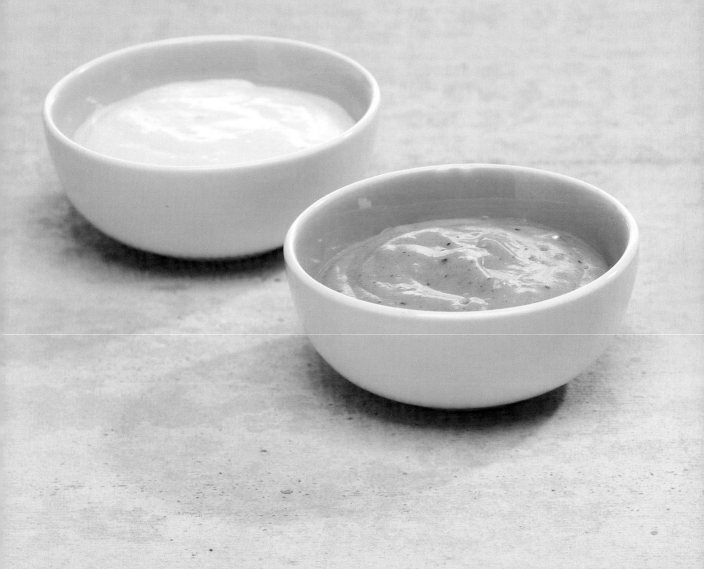

# Gluten-free Teriyaki Sauce

## Makes about 1 cup (250 mL)

Make your own gluten-free teriyaki sauce and serve it with beef or chicken dishes. Mirin and sake also add a great flavour to recipes on their own.

1/3 cup (75 mL) gluten-free light soy sauce

1/3 cup (75 mL) mirin

1/3 cup (75 mL) sake

1/2 tsp (2 mL) sugar

Combine all ingredients in a small pot. Simmer on medium, stirring until sugar is dissolved. Reduce heat to low. Simmer, uncovered, for 6 to 8 minutes until sauce is slightly thickened. Store sauce, covered, in fridge for 2 to 3 months.

*1/2 cup: 111 Calories; 0 g Total Fat (0 g Mono, 0 g Poly, 0 g Sat); 0 mg Cholesterol; 9 g Carbohydrate; 0 g Fibre; 6 g Protein; 1878 mg Sodium*

# Hollandaise Sauce

## Makes about 2 cups

You can never have enough of this creamy and tart sauce. This recipe has a little bit of a kick with the addition of cayenne and mustard. Use it over Eggs Benedict or any vegetable dish.

4 egg yolks (large), fork-beaten, room temperature

1/2 cup (125 mL) butter, melted

1/2 cup (125 mL) water

3 Tbsp (45 mL) lemon juice

1/2 tsp (2 mL) salt

1/2 tsp (2 mL) prepared mustard

1/8 tsp (0.5 mL) cayenne pepper

Combine egg yolks, butter and water in top of double boiler or heatproof bowl set over 1/2 cup (125 mL) simmering water. Cook, stirring constantly with whisk, until thickened. Remove from heat.

Add remaining 4 ingredients, stirring until well mixed. Serve hot.

*1 cup: 522 Calories; 55 g Total Fat (16 g Mono, 3 g Poly, 32 g Sat); 542 mg Cholesterol; 3 g Carbohydrate; 0 g Fibre; 6 g Protein; 940 mg Sodium*

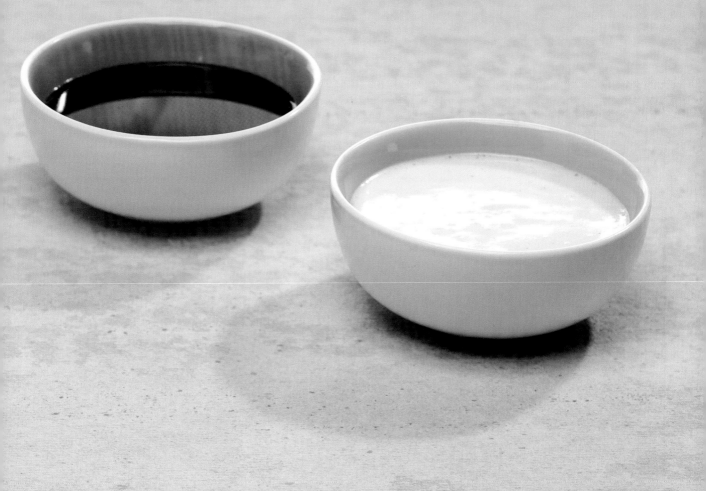

# Index

**A**

Apples, Donna's Turnips and, 146
Asian Pork Stew, 110

**B**

Béchamel Sauce, 154
Beef
  Goulash, 52
  Pot Pie, 66
  Stew, 50
  Stock, Classic, 34
  Stroganoff, 54
  Teriyaki, 64
  Wellington Supreme, 56
Bread Sticks, Garlic, 24
Breaded
  Lemon Chicken Breasts, 86
  Pan-fried Trout, 106
Broccoli Quiche, Crustless, 132
Brown Meat Gravy, 154
Bruschetta, 16
Burgers
  Chicken, 84
  Walnut Lentil, 134

**C**

Caesar Salad, 44
Cakes, Green Onion, 18
Calzones, Veggie, 136
Casserole
  Creamy Turkey, 96
  Potato Leek, 122
  Quinoa, 128
Cheddar Spritz, Spicy, 10
Chickpea Masala with
  Garlic Bread, 138

Chicken
  Breasts, Breaded Lemon, 86
  Burgers, 84
  Cordon Bleu, 76
  Curried, 82
  Drumsticks with
  Sweet Potato Fries, 80
  Fingers, 78
  Fried, 88
  Pie, 90
  Soup, Classic, 32
  Stew with Rice, 72
Chili Con Carne in a Bread Bowl, 68
Chris's Frittata Tarts, 30
Clam Chowder, 36
Classic
  Beef Stock, 34
  Chicken Soup, 32
Coq au Vin, 74
Corn Dogs, 20
Cornbread, 150
Creamy Turkey Casserole, 96
Crustless Broccoli Quiche, 132
Curried Chicken, 82
Curry Cream Shrimp, 102

**D**

Donna's Turnips and Apples, 146
Drumsticks, Chicken, with
  Sweet Potato Fries, 80

**F**

Falafel and Pita Bread, 130
Fish
  and Chips, 100
  Sticks, 98
Focaccia, 22
Fried Chicken, 88
Frittata Tarts, Chris's, 30

**G**

Garlic Bread
  Chickpea Masala with, 138
  Sticks, 24
Gluten-free Teriyaki Sauce, 154
Gravy, Brown Meat, 154
Green Onion Cakes, 18
Goulash, Beef, 52

**H**

Hollandaise Sauce, 156

**K**

Koenigsberger Klopse, 62

**L**

Lamb Chops, Rosemary, 126
Lasagna, 70
Lemon
  Chicken Breasts, Breaded, 86
  Pork Wrap, 124
Lentil Burgers, Walnut, 134

**M**

Mac 'n' Cheese, 140
Masala, Chickpea, with
  Garlic Bread, 138
Meatballs, Spaghetti and, 60
Meatloaf, 58
Minestrone, 38
Mushroom Soup, Wild, 40

**P**

Pan-fried Trout, Breaded, 106
Pasta
  Salad, Tuna, 48
  Scallops and Shrimp, 108

Perogies, 116
Pie, Chicken, 90
Pilaf, 144
Pita Bread, Falafel and, 130
Pizza Pockets, 118
Pommes de Terre an Gratin, 153
Pork
  Stew, Asian, 110
  Sweet and Sour, 114
  Wrap, Lemon, 124
Pot Pie, Beef, 66
Potato
  Leek Casserole, 122
  Pancakes, 28
  Pommes de Terre au Gratin, 153
Poultry Stuffing, 148
Puff Shrimp with Orange
  Ginger Sauce, 14

**Q**

Quiche
  Broccoli, Crustless, 132
  Lorraine, 120
Quinoa
  Casserole, 128
  Salad, 42

**R**

Ravioli, Tortellini and, 92
Rosemary Lamb Chops, 126

**S**

Salad
  Caesar, 44
  Quinoa, 42
  Tuna Pasta, 48
  Waldorf, 46
Scallops and Shrimp Pasta, 108
Schnitzel, Wiener, 112
Shrimp
  Curry Cream, 102
  Pasta, Scallops and, 108
  Puff, with Orange Ginger Sauce, 14
  Tartlets, 12
Slow Sweet and Spicy
  Seafood Stew, 104
Spaetzle, 142
Spaghetti and Meatballs, 60
Spicy Cheddar Spritz, 10
Stew
  Asian Pork, 110
  Beef, 50
  Chicken, with Rice, 72
  Slow Sweet and Spicy Seafood, 104
Stroganoff, Beef, 54
Stuffing, Poultry, 148
Sweet and Sour Pork
Sweet Potato Fries, Chicken
  Drumsticks with, 80

**T**

Teriyaki
  Beef, 64
  Sauce, Gluten-free, 156
Thanksgiving Turkey Dinner, 94
Tortellini and Ravioli, 92
Tortillas and Dip, 26
Trout, Breaded Pan-fried, 106
Tuna Pasta Salad, 48
Turkey
  Casserole, Creamy, 96
  Dinner, Thanksgiving, 94
Turnips and Apples, Donna's, 146

**V**

Veggie Calzones, 136

**W**

Waldorf Salad, 46
Walnut Lentil Burgers, 134
Wiener Schnitzel, 112
Wild Mushroom Soup, 40
Wrap, Lemon Pork, 124

# Acknowledgements

The book you are holding and reading, like any good thing in life, is the product of many great people coming together and embarking on a journey to create something special. The vibrant energies that I've encountered in putting this book together are many and are frankly quite amazing.

The many thousands of customers that I had the pleasure of meeting over many years as founder and former owner of internationally renowned gluten-free manufacturer Kinnikinnick Foods Inc. are the main driving force for this book. To the many business partners and colleagues in the gluten-free food-manufacturing world, I applaud you for providing more and more great-tasting gluten-free products.

Thank you to all the absolutely brilliant people at Company's Coming whose creativity, vision and enthusiasm extend beyond any book. I had the honour of meeting and working with so many of you, too many to list all of you. To name a few, I would like to thank Linda Dobos for their help in preparing the recipes for the photo sessions, and for noticing that maybe that 4 Tbsp of baking powder should possibly read 4 tsp. I know you, the reader, will appreciate this.

Thank you Ashley Billey for her countless hours of helping with the preparation of the recipes and her absolutely amazing food styling skills. She can make a banana peel look like a crème brûlée.

Thank you to my main photographer Sandy Weatherall for her incredible vision, her desire for perfection, her creative focus and unsurpassed photography skills. She makes me want to bite into the book.

Thank you Jordan Allan and Nancy Foulds, the editors who put up with my Germanized English and put my creative vision into a printable format.

I also want to thank *you*. Yes, I mean *you*, the one reading this right now. I like to thank you personally for the part you played in creating this book. The time we have together is very special and valuable. Know that I specifically express my gratitude to your contribution and that I have been waiting here in these words, just for you to connect. Have an awesome day!

I like to take this moment to thank the Earth and all the loving energies that bring us wonderful food and nutritious ingredients for our enjoyment. I have had wonderful opportunities in my life to know where my food is coming from, where it was grown, how it was grown and, in many cases, who grew it, the farmer or processor. I am blessed to know of the value of food and diet to maintain proper health, while at the same time having countless hours of fun socializing and connecting with friends and family through cooking and meal preparation.

Thank you for cooking with me!